LYMINGTON.

Considered solely as a watering-place, Lymington has little that can recommend it; but viewed with all its accompaniments, it would be unjust to deny that it has claims to attention which few situations can boast. Its vicinity to the Isle of Wight, with which it maintains a daily communication, and the various beauties of the New Forest, on the verge of which it lies, are attractions that cannot be overlooked.

Lymington is eighteen miles from Southampton, the road to which is through the middle of the New Forest, the most delightful in England, and about 95 miles from London. It stands about a mile from the channel which separates England from the Isle of Wight, on the brow and declivity of a gentle hill; a circumstance which adds to its cleanliness, and increases its salubrity. It consists principally of one long street, with a descent towards the quay: the buildings are in general decent, and some of them rather elegant. Many of the houses enjoy delightful perspectives of the Channel and the Isle of Wight, with its bold aspiring cliffs. The Angel Inn, in point of size and elegance, can accommodate several families, and has attached to it an elegant assembly-room. The town-hall, which is a very neat building, has also occasionally been used for the latter purpose. The other houses of public entertainment are also very respectable.

At the bottom of the town runs the Lymington river, which, when the tide is at its height, presents a fine extensive sheet of water; ships of 200 or 300 tons burthen can commodiously lie within a few feet of the quay, and formerly vessels of 500 tons could have done the same; but the injudicious measure of throwing a causeway across the river, to the north of the town, has been the means of permitting the mud to accumulate in the river; this, however, is expected will be remedied, a new bridge, with proper flood-gates, having been erected, which, by retaining the back-water till the tide has ebbed, will soon clear out, and cleanse the channel. The port is appendant to that of Southampton, the jurisdiction of which is very extensive.

Lymington has but little commerce: its chief import is coals; and export, salt, which is its only manufacture of any consequence, and this is greatly on the decline. Still, however, various kinds, both medicinal and culinary, of excellent quality, are made at the works contiguous to the town. This manufacture appears to be of very great antiquity. In 1147 a tythe of the Lymington salt was given to the monks of Quarr abbey, in the Isle of Wight. Not half a century ago fifty thousand pounds were paid annually into the exchequer for duty; but this manufacture is now undersold in different parts of the kingdom, and in consequence the trade here has greatly fallen off.*

Lymington has two sets of baths, one at the bottom of the town, the other about half a mile from it. These have lately been made very convenient, and the proprietors have endeavoured to pay every attention to the comfort of the bathers; and as these baths can be used at any time of the day without being obliged to pay regard to the time of the tide, they are particularly suited to the convenience of invalids. The immense body of water which passes in through the Needles, and the flow of the river water being restrained by the flood-gates, during the whole of each tide,

* The salt here is made in the following manner: The sea-water is first pumped into shallow square pits dug in the earth, called pans. In these it is exposed to the heat of the sun till it becomes seven times more saline by evaporation than it was in its original state. It is then pumped into flat iron pans, eight or ten feet square, and as many inches deep; and in these the brine is boiled over a fierce fire, till nothing but pure salt remains. When this has been drained in proper vessels, it is fit for use.

renders bathing here equally as salutary as at any other bathing-place.

The reasonableness of this place, joined to the beauty of its situation, draws to it a considerable number of stationary company during the season, and as it lies so near Southampton, and the Isle of Wight, it receives shoals of flying visitors from both.

We doubt not but it will be acceptable to our readers to learn, that Dr. Marshall, celebrated for his vaccine tour through the south of Europe, and who resided at Paris during the interval of peace, and whose skilful attendance upon them, many will recollect with pleasure, has fixed his residence here.

Lymington is a very ancient place,* and according to tradition, it has been three times sacked and burnt by the French. There is reason indeed to suppose, that its ancient church perished in one of those desolating visits, as its site may be traced on the north of the present town, near a place called Broad-lane. The oldest part of the existing church does not appear of higher antiquity than the reign of Henry VI. nor does it contain any thing remarkable, except a curious notice in the register for the year 1736, that "Samuel Baldwin, esq. sojourner in this parish, was immersed without the Needles, in Scratcher's Bay, *sans ceremonie*, May 20th." It is said that this singular mode of burial was in compliance with the will of the deceased, and that his motive was to prevent his wife from "dancing over his grave," which she had, it seems, frequently threatened to do, in case she survived him. This church is dependant on Boldre, the vicar of which has the right of nomination to the cure.

Though Lymington was a borough in the reign of Edward III. and sent members to parliament in that of Elizabeth, it was not incorporated till the reign of James I. who vested the right of electing representa-

* Nearly two hundred pounds weight of coins of the Lower Empire were found here in 1744; an incontestible proof that the Romans must have resided on the spot.

tives in the mayor and burgesses, in whom it still remains.

Except reading, for which the libraries furnish a tolerable invitation, walking, riding, and sailing, there are few amusements at Lymington which can engage the gay, or relieve the languor of the old. The botanist, however, will find in this vicinity treasures worthy his observation. In a black bog on the right of the road to Southampton, a little beyond the third mile-stone from Lymington, the writer of this found, in 1802, the narthecium ossifragum, or Lancastrian asphodel, which was never known to grow so far south, the drosera or sun-dew, with several other curious plants. In short, this neighbourhood has never been accurately examined; and therefore it promises to furnish new stores.

RIDES AND WALKS ROUND LYMINGTON.

Every part of the New Forest has its appropriate beauties, and will be visited by persons of taste with rapture; but as we naturally excurse thither from Southampton, only contiguous objects will be noticed in this place.

Brockenhurst is a pleasant village, lying in a vale adorned with the most charming scenery. The view from the church-yard, which stands on an eminence, is fine as well as extensive. At the entrance of the church-yard is a remarkably large oak, and also a stately yew, fifteen feet in girt, and upwards of sixty feet high. Brockenhurst-house commands a fine forest view; and Watcombe-house, in the same neighbourhood, will ever be interesting in the eye of humanity, for having been the residence of the philanthropic Howard: but it was entirely pulled down upwards of seven years ago. The spot on which it stood can only be traced by a farm-house, and a dairy.

Vicar's-hill, the late residence of the amiable and ingenious Mr. Gilpin, late vicar of Boldre, will also be viewed with more than common interest; and in itself it is a charming situation, which was much improved by the taste of that worthy divine.

About a mile from Lymington are the traces of a Roman camp, known by the name of Buckland Rings, or Castle Field. Its form is an oblong square, rounded at the corners, the area being about 200 paces in length and 170 in breadth. The works are nearly entire, except towards the river. It was defended by three ramparts, and as many ditches.

In visiting Hurst Castle, we pass the pleasant villa of Capt. Payton, called Priestlands. Hurst castle stands near the extremity of a tongue of land, which projects two miles into the sea, leaving a channel of not more than a mile broad between it and the Isle of Wight. The castle was built by Henry VIII. about the year 1539, and consists of a round tower, fortified by semicircular bastions. Here Charles I. was brought prisoner from the Isle of Wight, by Colonel Corbet, and kept till General Harrison carried him to London, previously to his unfortunate end. Here, too, Mr. Atkinson, a popish priest, was immured thirty years, for exercising his office in England contrary to law. He bore his long confinement with exemplary patience, and died in the seventy-fourth year of his age, in the reign of George I. A small garrison is constantly kept in Hurst castle.

CHRISTCHURCH.

This ancient sea-port town lies twelve miles from Lymington, and derives its name from a large collegiate church built here in the time of the West Saxons. This church is a venerable and stately pile, upwards of 300 feet in length, and contains many objects well worthy of observation. Around it are some vestiges of a monastery.

Christchurch is a borough, the right of returning two members to serve in parliament being in the corporation. It is a pleasant town, and has a large manufactory, which employs a number of children in making watch-chains. The place is also famous for a fine salmon fishery.

Since sea-bathing has become the rage, Christchurch has aspired to the same privileges as its neighbours; and certainly its claims, in this respect, are well-founded. The shore, which is about two miles from the down, is composed of a good hard sand, free from stones. Here is a small hamlet called Muddiford, where are kept seven bathing-machines, and a warm sea-bath, provided by Mr. Beamister.

The King's Arms Inn and Hotel at Christchurch, kept by Mr. Humby, is an excellent house of accommodation, and commands a beautiful and uninterrupted prospect of the Isle of Wight and the Needles. This house, which is unquestionably one of the first inns in the kingdom, was built about three years since, by the Right Hon. George Rose, for the accommodation of visitors resorting hither for the purpose of bathing, till they can be provided with lodgings near the sea at Muddiford, or in the town.

The roads to Christchurch are very good, and afford beautiful views in all directions. From Southampton through Lyndhurst, across the forest, the distance is 24 miles; from Salisbury, by Fording-bridge and Ringwood, 27 miles; and from hence to Weymouth, through Winborne and Blandford, 46 miles.

HIGH CLIFF.

The late Earl of Bute having taken a fancy to this place, erected a magnificent house in the neighbourhood, on a lofty eminence, which commands one of the most beautiful sea-views in the kingdom, partly from the proximity of the Isle of Wight on one side, and partly from the opening into the Channel on the other. To this place his lordship would often retire from his noble seat of Luton, in Bedfordshire, for the express purpose of obtaining a sound sleep, which he declared he could find here, when it was to be had no where else. High Cliff, the name of his seat, now very much reduced in point of size, is the property of J. Penleaze, Esq.

In the cliff on which this house is built, various fossils have been found, a valuable collection of which was presented to the British Museum by the late Mr. Brander, who possessed a seat in the neighbourhood. There are several other pleasant seats near Christchurch: and Mr. Rose has recently erected a pretty cottage in a very simple yet elegant stile, in which he has been imitated by Lady Stuart.

On the other side of Lymington, Walthampton, the seat of Sir Harry Burrard Neale; Beaulieu Abbey, still venerable in its ruins; and numerous other beautiful scenes and situations, well deserve the tourist's attention.

MALVERN.

Strongly impressed with an idea, which observation on the spot has confirmed, that the Malvern hills, on account of the salubrity of the air, are not less restorative to health than the Wells, we shall begin with the former and advise visitors and invalids who resort to this place to do the same.

The Malvern chain lies in the three counties of Worcester, Gloucester, and Hereford, but principally in the former. Before it, on the east, spreads an extensive plain of luxuriant fertility; on the west, or Herefordshire side, the country is more broken and uneven, but in general not less prolific.

These hills extend about nine miles in length, and from one or two miles and upwards in breadth. The highest parts are those distinguished by the name of the Herefordshire and Worcestershire beacons, which are about four miles distant from each other; the former rising about 1260 feet, and the latter about 1300 feet, above the level of the plain.

Malvern hills consist of various strata, chiefly granite, a silecious substance of a grey colour, mixed with red veins; it resists acids, and takes a good polish. They contain also a considerable quantity of quartz, and a great variety of calcareous, mineral, and argillaceous substances, detached in masses, or deposited in veins in the superincumbent gravel. The most remarkable of these productions is a large mass of ore,* lying on the summit of the hill, about a mile to the southward of the village of Great Malvern. This being ponderous, was supposed to contain some kind of metal; but, from repeated expe-

* Among this ore has been found that curious production the asbestus or amianthus; and on another part of the hills a quantity of spar formed in hexagonal chrystalline figures.

Page 300

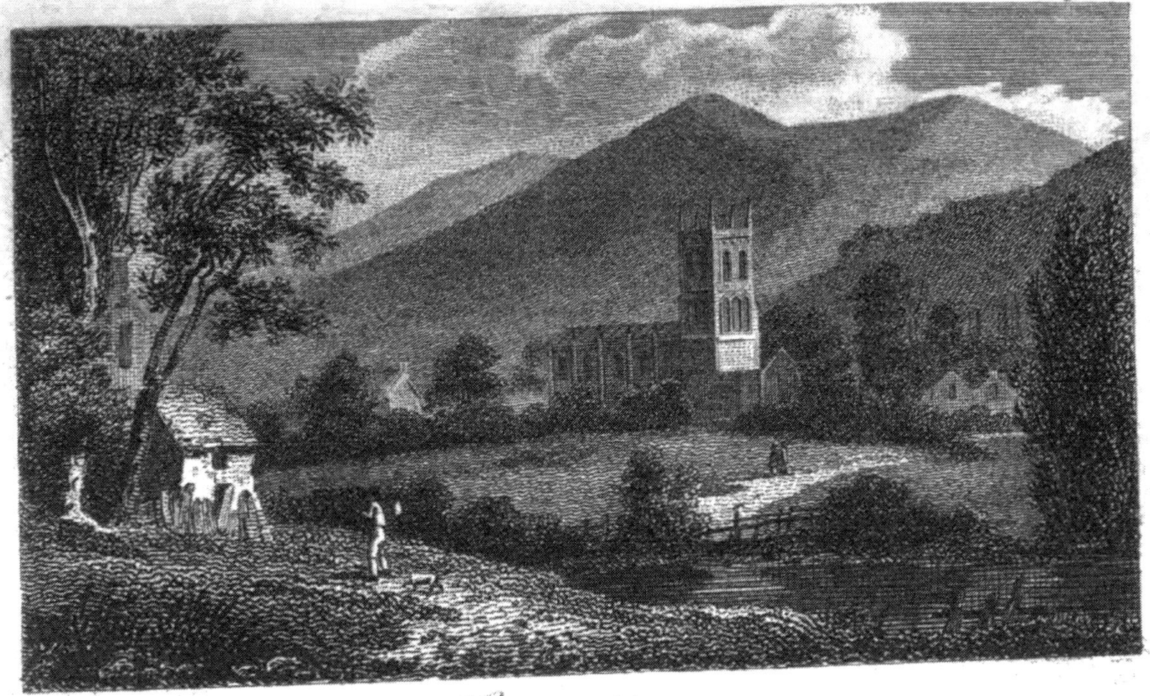

Great Malvern.

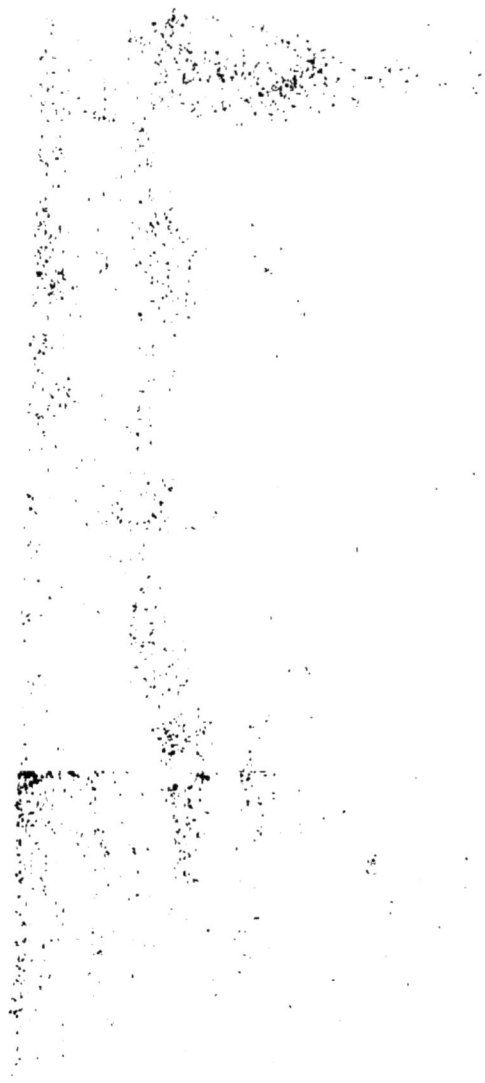

riments, it is found to be a kind of mica, not fusible by any known process. It is probable, however, that in the bowels of the hill are some valuable metallic substances. The western declivity contains a bed of limestone, in which many fossil substances are discovered.

The more elevated parts of Malvern hills not being susceptible of cultivation, are uninclosed, producing chiefly gorse and fern, with a short sweet herbage, very grateful to sheep. The digitalis, and other beautiful and rare plants, grow here in the utmost luxuriance. The Alpine heights of Malvern are favourable for the production of vegetables that delight in a cold exposure, and the bottoms of the hills have likewise their appropriate plants.

On the Herefordshire Beacon are the remains of an ancient camp, consisting of a double intrenchment, the outermost about half a mile in circumference. The avenues or passes are still to be seen, and the greatest part is in fine preservation; but whether the work is Roman, British, or Saxon, has not been determined.

About a mile and a half further to the southward, on a protuberance of the hill, are the remains of another camp, consisting of only a single ditch; and on the declivity of the Herefordshire Beacon is a cave cut in the rock, about ten feet long, six broad, and seven high, of rude workmanship, and unknown origin.

About fifty years ago a considerable quantity of silver coin was found on the west side of those hills: but the most singular discovery was that of a crown or coronet of gold set with precious stones, which was dug up near one of the castrametations in 1650. The cottager who found this valuable relic, sold it for no more than 37*l.*; but it appears that the jewels only fetched 1500*l.* and that the gold was worth about 1000*l.* more. This singular curiosity falling into the hands of avaricious persons, was destroyed before the learned were apprised of the discovery.

Some suppose it to have been the diadem of a British prince slain in this vicinity.

On the declivity of Malvern, in the parish of Eastnor, are the ruins of Bransil castle, of which but little now remains. It appears to have been of great antiquity the site is the property of lord Somers.

HOLY-WELL, &c.

A variety of springs issue from the Malvern hills, of various qualities, according to the substances they are impregnated with; but that which has been for several ages reputed peculiarly salutary, and has obtained the name of Holy-well, rises on the east side of the hill, half way up, about two miles from Great Malvern, and one from Little Malvern, both in the county of Worcester.

According to the late eminent Dr. Wall, of Worcester, the water of this spring "does not contain any uncombined vitriolic acid, nor any volatile alkali, nor any metallic salt; but is slightly impregnated with fixed air, some common air, some selenites, and a little unneutralised calcareous earth. "Hence," he observes, "the principal virtue of Malvern water must depend on its extreme purity, assisted by the fixed air which it contains."

Dr. Johnstone, another distinguished physician in Worcester, lately deceased, agrees in the above analysis, except that he could not find the Holy-well water contained any fixed air; but from his own experience declared, that he had found it beneficial in scrophulous cases, cutaneous eruptions, and nephritic complaints; and farther remarked, "that the temperate warmth of the air, and the great purity of the water at Malvern, induced him to consider that place peculiarly favourable for patients afflicted with nervous disorders, or inclined to consumptions, especially in the summer and autumnal months."

In cancerous complaints, old ulcers, glandular obstructions, and other complaints for which Malvern water has been prescribed, drinking, lotion, and bathing, according to circumstances, must be used. Early rising, exercise on foot or horseback, with temperance, must be combined with the water; and if the former are regularly pursued and observed, the effects of the latter will be a consequence rather than a cause.

The source of the Holy-well is secured by a convenient erection, containing a bath and other accommodations; and at a small distance is a large and commodious lodging-house, capable of receiving a considerable number of people, who dine at a public table, and live very sociably together. Here is also a billiard-room to amuse them in bad weather; but such is the romantic situation of the place, and the indescribable beauty of the landscapes, that strangers for some time will feel little disposition to ennui, if they enjoy their eye-sight. Company, however, seldom stay long in this place; but there is a constant succession from Cheltenham, and many other parts of the kingdom, during the summer season.

About April, May, and June, when the fruit-trees are in blossom, no situation in the kingdom can afford a richer prospect than this. It seems the very centre of Pomona's reign, who, if she erects her throne on the summit of Malvern, may behold all the glories of her train. In winter this situation is too much exposed to the cold to be agreeable; and therefore we may suppose the goddess, and those who are fond of swelling her court, retire to milder regions.

Near the Well-house, as this hotel is called, are several delightful walks, which by a winding ascent lead to the summit of the hill, from whence may be discerned Monmouthshire, Radnorshire, Herefordshire, Brecknockshire, Staffordshire, Shropshire, Gloucestershire, Worcestershire, Oxfordshire, and Warwickshire; some of them appearing uniform from the distance, and others beautifully diversified by nature and art. The cities of Gloucester, Worcester, and Hereford, are visible, with several market towns; and, with the assistance of a glass, nearly a hundred churches. The beautiful city of Worcester in particular, though more than eight miles off, appears in all its pride, from every point on the eastern side of the hills.

RIDES, &c.

There are several delightful rides about the Malvern hills. The Worcester road towards Ledbury, skirting the hill with gradual ascent, till it enters a pass near Little Malvern, unfolds many beautiful prospects as we advance. The luxuriant appearance of the proximity finely contrasts with the sterile aspect of the Malvern chain; the one presents nature in her gayest dress; the other nature in her naked and romantic features.

At the distance of two miles is another public road over the hill, cut through the Wytch. This is so precipitous that it is seldom used for carriages; and a person who is unaccustomed to such elevations, grows giddy as he looks down from the summit on the immense champaign below. The valetudinary will likewise perceive some degree of fainting on reaching the bottom, from the sudden alteration in the pressure of the air.

The late Sir Hildebrand Jacob, bart. was at a considerable expence in making a road, by which carriages may be taken round the south part of the hill; and it is impossible to find a ride that presents more picturesque views than this. In short, on the Malvern hills the very air we breathe is invigorating; it produces an appetite and exhilarates the spirits, while epidemical diseases are seldom known within these precincts. "We sometimes want victuals," said a poor cottager to the writer of this, "but we never want a doctor:" and perhaps he spoke truth; yet, notwithstanding the general purity of the water, there are petrifying springs on the west side of the hills, which being used for culinary purposes, sometimes occasion wens, or strumous swellings of the maxillary glands.

GREAT MALVERN.

The genteel village of Great Malvern, where the greatest part of the company reside, though two miles distant from the Holy-well, is distant about 120 miles from London, eight from Worcester, and 22 from Cheltenham. It is charmingly situated on the eastern declivity of the hill, and consists of about fifty houses, interspersed with gardens, orchards, and plantations. Most of the buildings are neat, and, except those belonging to individuals of fortune, let wholly or in part during the season, and sometimes on high terms. Here the aspect of the hill is peculiarly striking, and forms a wonderful contrast with the adjoining country, where cultivation and fertility are the predominant features in the landscape.

In a dimple of the hill, about a quarter of a mile above the church, rises St. Anne's Well, which is equally pure and salutary with the Holy-well, though less used. The ascent to it is by a zig-zag foot-path.

In the meadows below the village is a chalybeate spring, once highly celebrated, but now in a great measure neglected.

The Crown Hotel, at Great Malvern, is well calculated for the reception of company. It stands near the centre of the village, and commands from its windows variegated and extensive prospects.

Great Malvern was famous for its monastery, founded about the year 1083, but few vestiges of it now remain, except the church, which being purchased by the inhabitants, was rendered parochial. This is still a magnificent structure, being 171 feet long and 63 broad, with an embattled and pinnacled tower, springing from the centre, 124 feet high. The style of architecture is rather airy, considering the time when it was erected; and the painted glass in the windows was once greatly admired. It represented many scenes from scripture history;

but time and neglect have left them mutilated and broken, though enough remains to give an idea of their former beauty.

Several parts of the choir are ornamented with a tesselated pavement, containing the coats of arms of many ancient and noble families. The tombs and monumental inscriptions are numerous, and some of them very ancient. The inscription on Walcher, the second prior of Malvern, which was discovered in 1711, is dated 1135.

LITTLE MALVERN.

Little Malvern, which forms a separate parish at the distance of more than three miles from Great Malvern, lies in a recumbent slope near the entrance of the great recess in the hill. It was once a considerable village, but now contains only five or six houses. Here likewise was a monastery, founded about the year 1171. Before the Conquest, all the surrounding country was a wilderness, thick set with trees, to which some hermits retired; and their number increasing, they agreed to assume the monastic habit, and to live according to the order of St. Benedict. From this circumstance arose the convent both at Great and Little Malvern.

The church of the latter, which is now ruinous, was rebuilt in 1482, by John Alcock, bishop of Worcester, and was adorned with windows of painted glass, of which little now remains.

Near the church is an antique building on the site of the ancient monastery, which, viewed either from the hill above, or the plain below, is the object of admiration, for its romantic and sequestered situation.

The country on the west side of the Malvern hills is thick-studded with plantations of apple and pear-trees. On the east, or Worcestershire side, was a large tract, lately inclosed, which constituted the ancient Malvern chase, formerly well stocked with deer, and belonging to the crown. Edward I. gave it to Gilbert de Clare, Earl of Gloucester, between whom and the bishop of Hereford, a dispute soon arose respecting the western boundary. To mark this, a great ditch was drawn along the ridge of the hill, which is still in many parts in good preservation.

SEATS, &C.

The picturesque beauty and healthiness of the surrounding country have induced several persons of distinction to fix their residence in this district. Hope End, the seat of Sir Henry Tempest, bart. lies about three miles from Malvern Wells, and is a spacious mansion; the grounds are remarkably well wooded and diversified.

The villa of Mr. Brydges, in the same neighbourhood, is pleasantly situate, at the foot of a woody eminence. From Brand-Green Lodge, distant about a mile from Malvern Wells, and standing on an elevation 500 feet above the plain, is a fine view of the camp, which has already been mentioned.

At Eastnor, which is also on the western side of Malvern, and four miles from the Wells, is Castleditch, the seat of Lord Somers. The greatest part of the building is ancient, but there are some elegant modern additions. Being built on a flat, this house loses the charm of distant prospects; but it possesses so many beauties within the appendant domains, that they are less required.

Near the southern extremity of Malvern hills is Bromsberow-place, a handsome building with agreeable accompaniments and enchanting prospects.

Blackmore Park, in Worcestershire, about two miles from the Wells, is a modern and elegant structure, but possesses no extensive views.

Madresfield, the seat of the Lygon family, is an antique, but neat building, and commands delightful views of the Malvern hills, from which it is distant about four miles.

Crome Court, the splendid seat of the Earl of Coventry, is within an easy morning ride of Malvern, and deserves a minute inspection. It was built under the direction of the celebrated Capability Brown.

The beautiful and genteel village of Powic, about six miles from Great Malvern, and two from Worcester, is an assemblage of rural villas, each of which has its appropriate charms.

No stranger, from whatever part of the country he comes to Malvern, will miss the opportunity of visiting Worcester, one of the most elegant cities in the kingdom for its size. The cathedral is peculiarly beautiful: and in it will be seen the tombs of the worthless King John; of the youthful Prince Arthur, eldest son of Henry VII.; of the beautiful Countess of Salisbury, whose garter is said to have given rise to the most illustrious order of knighthood in the world; and of the pious and patriotic Hough, once bishop of this diocese, whose monument, by Roubilliac, is one of the most expressive and elegant pieces of sculpture which that great artist ever produced.

The subsequent elegant lines, written by a lady at Malvern Wells, in 1801, are for the first time given to the public, and will form a pleasing epilogue to this article.

Where Malvern rears her sky-capp'd head,
    And smiling Health has fix'd her court,
Where purest streams their blessings shed,
    And balmy zephyrs, laughing sport;

I often wander forth at eve,
    To view the soft retreat of day;
The tranquil shades my mind relieve,
    As night unfolds her cloak of grey.

Then, where no footsteps mark the hill,
    Or sounds obtrusive strike the ear,
Save the low murmur of the rill
    That fills Hygeia's fountain near,

I woo thee, Hope, "sweet child of heaven!"
  And press thee fondly to my breast:
For, ah! to thee the power is given
  To soothe e'en Misery to rest!

O, never more my bosom leave!
  Too long the prey of fell Despair;
Still with delusive tales—deceive——
  Still, smiling, chase away my care!

Bid drooping Fancy live anew;
  Her pencil guide, with fairy art:
Tint her soft scenes with golden hue,
  And let the sunshine reach my heart!

E. C. S.

MARGATE.

Margate, conveniently stationed in respect to the metropolis for conveyance by water or land, and delightfully situated on the populous and finely cultivated Isle of Thanet, is always enlivened by a more numerous company than any other sea-bathing place. The Hoys, which sail every tide from Billingsgate, are cheap, and sometimes agreeable and rapid conveyances; but as the distance by land is only 73 miles, the roads good, and the vehicles numerous and certain, most persons, ladies especially, prefer the passage by land.

DESCRIPTION OF THE ISLE OF THANET.

The Isle of Thanet, at the eastern extremity of Kent, is about nine miles long, and five broad. It is separated from the county by the river Stour on the southern side, and by the water called the Nethergong on the western; and is surrounded by the sea on the northern and eastern sides, along which the cliffs extend from Gore End on the south, to Cliff End on the east.

Thanet is divided into two capital manors, Minster and Monkton, and contains eleven parishes; but only seven churches have withstood the levelling hand of time. The chalk cliffs on the north and east parts are generally pretty high, in some places abounding with fossils; and under them occasionally have been found large pieces of amber, particularly after a storm and a convulsion of the cliff. Through these cliffs the inhabitants have cut several openings to the sea, for the conveniency of fishing, and of procuring manure from the beach; and these in former times they were obliged to secure, to prevent the predatory incursions of foreign enemies, who frequently landed here. Indeed, this island seems to derive its name from the

Page 304.

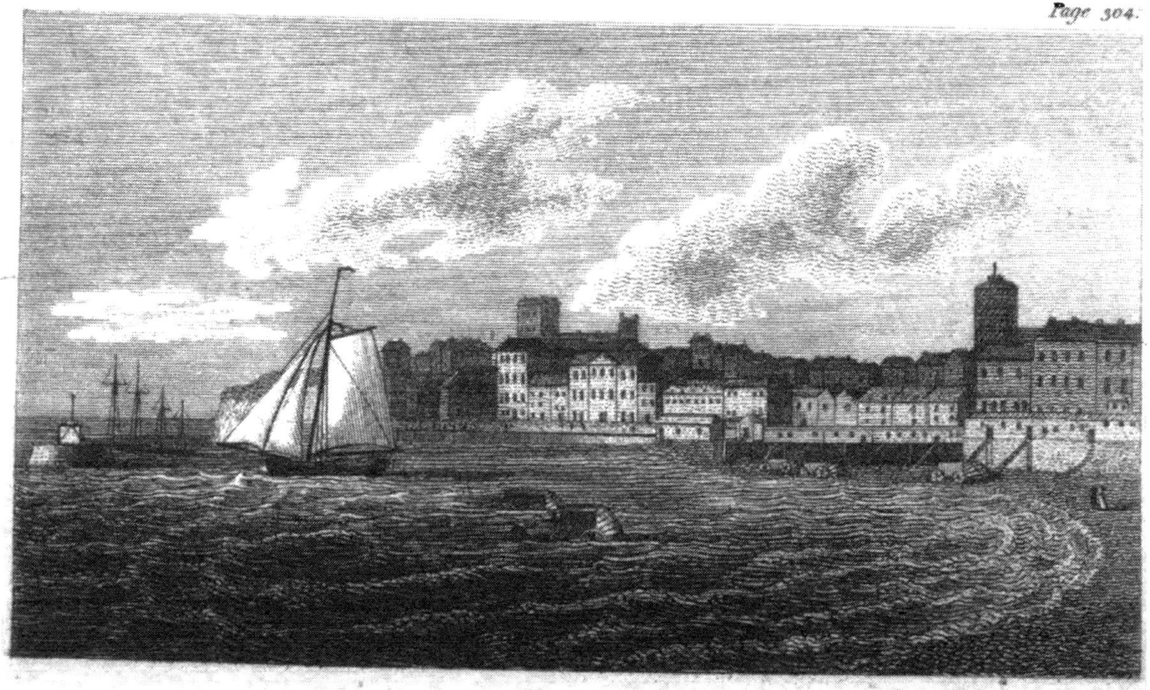

Margate.

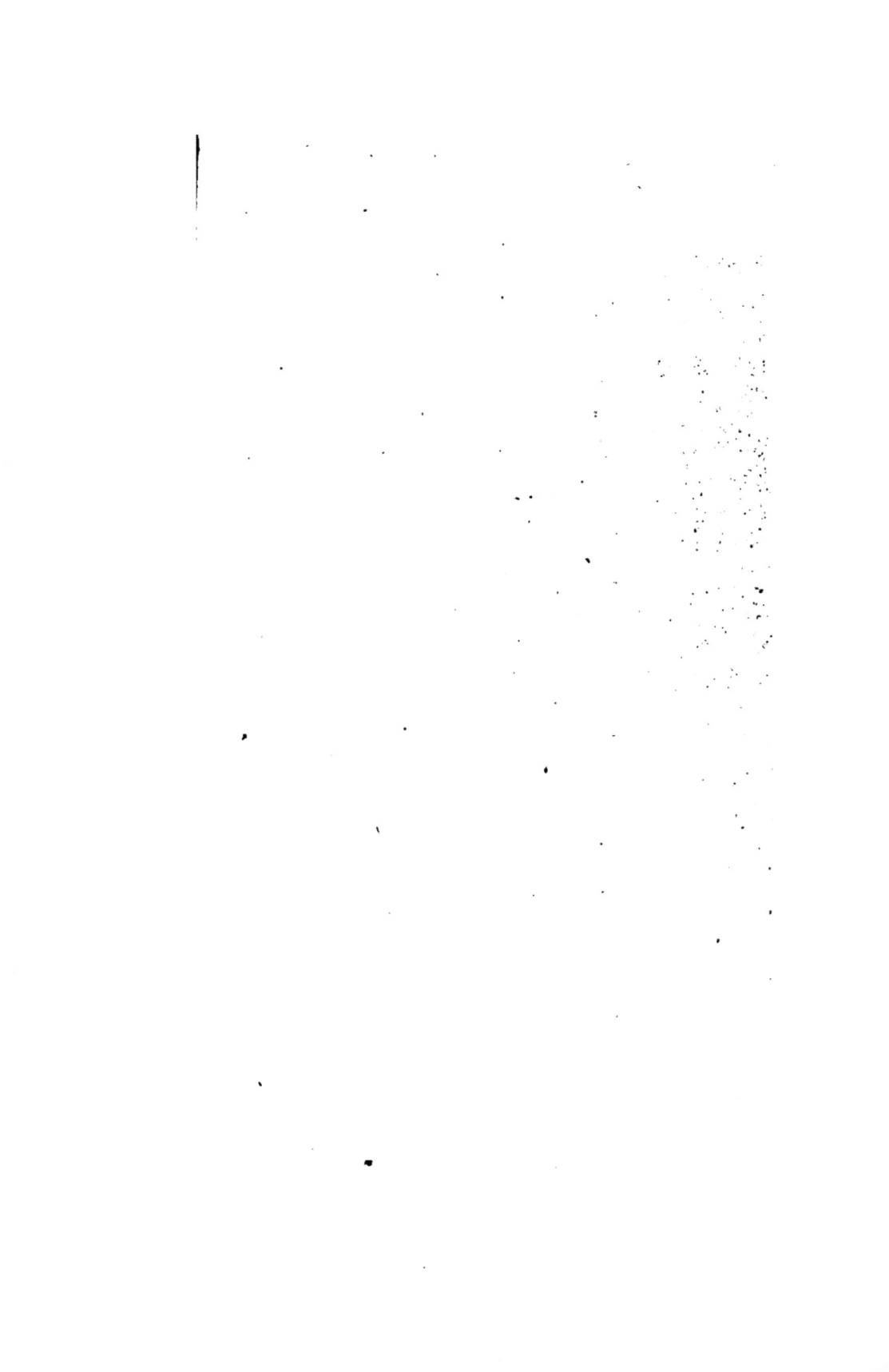

Saxon Tene, a fire, or beacon; of which it was necessary to keep up numbers, when the Danes and other pirates used to molest our coasts.

The general face of the country, except the marshland towards the south, is high and extremely rich, consisting of fertile corn lands intermixed with artificial grasses, mostly open and uninclosed; and the hamlets and cottages being generally built of chalk, as well as the boundary walls, the whole district has a cheerful aspect. Roads intersect it in every direction where communication can be wanted, so that almost every point is accessible; and the constant passing of vessels to and from the Medway and the Thames, gives the highest animation to the scene.

No situation can be more grateful in summer; but as the general aspect of Thanet is towards the north and east, and is totally unprotected by hedges or inclosures; during the colder months it is ungenial and forbidding to those who have been accustomed to more sheltered abodes. The inhabitants, however, except towards the marshes, seem as healthy and long-lived as in other places; and, in point of fertility, it is supposed that the produce of one year is equal to the consumption of three. Besides corn, vast quantities of canary-seed, and many esculent plants and roots, for the use of the London market, are raised here. Wet, as is common on chalky soils, is most favourable to its vegetation, and confirms the monkish proverb which says,

> "When England wrings
> The island sings."

The farms are generally large, and the occupiers intelligent and wealthy. They seem acquainted with the best modes of agriculture, and they do not till an ungrateful soil. Elm is the principal kind of timber produced here; but the bleak air from the sea is little propitious to any vegetable that outlives a single season Considering the extent of Thanet, the population is considerable, but there are few residents among them, above the rank of farmers and yeomanry. The greatest number of the inhabitants of the coasts are fishermen in general, and husbandmen on occasion: being an amphibious sort, equally skilled in holding the helm and the plough.

Thanet abounds with wild-fowl in severe winters. The bergander, or chenalopex, often frequents the marshes and waters; the nightingale constantly visits this island, and there are quails, partridges, hares, and rabbits; but the fox, badger, and otter, are seldom seen.

Several plants grow in this spot which may be considered as scarce and curious. Fennel is produced naturally, and in such abundance, that it is collected and sent to the London markets. Lemon and common thyme is also very plentiful; and, unfortunately for the farmers, the *brassica muralis*, or at least a variety of it, called here the stinkweed, from its fetid smell, begins to infest the lands. It was accidently propagated here by means of a shipwreck, and it will be difficult to eradicate it.

The hundred of Ringslow claims jurisdiction over such parts of this island as are not within that of the cinque-ports. These, however, extend their power over Margate, Ramsgate, and indeed the greatest part of the district.

The roads in Thanet are excellent, and the traveller finds no interruptions from turnpikes. The bottom being chalky, and the country pretty level, the roads are maintained at a small expence; but, from their multiplicity and frequent intersections, a stranger, without consulting the local map, will often be misled.

PASSAGE TO MARGATE.

But it is time to proceed to Margate, to which there are plenty of conveyances, both by sea and land. Post-chaises and stage-coaches present nothing particular, being the same in most parts of the kingdom, except that on this road the drivers of such vehicles, as well as their masters, are said to be characteristically impertinent and imposing; but a passage in the Margate-hoy, which, like the grave, levels all distinctions, is frequently so replete with whim, incident, and character, that it may be considered as a dramatic entertainment on the stage of the ocean. The fare being only 7*s*. for the common cabin; 9*s*. for the second, and 13*s*. for the state cabin, (including a duty of 1*s*. on each passenger), is a strong inducement for numbers to prefer this mode of traveling, though it cannot be recommended to persons of delicacy.

Here the high and low, rich and poor, the sick and sound, the gentleman and blackguard, are all jumbled together; and though there is much for the humourist to laugh at, there is more to offend the decent and well-bred. From Peter Pindar's ode to this vehicle take the following lines: the whole is a just picture of such a voyage.

Go, beauteous hoy, in safety every inch;
That storms should wreck thee, gracious heaven forbid!
Whether commanded by brave Captain Finch,
Or equally tremendous Captain Kidd:
Go with thy cargo—Margate town amuse,
And God preserve thy Christians and thy Jews!
  Soon as thou gett'st within the pier,
All Margate will be out, I trow,
  And people rush from far and near,
As if thou hadst wild beasts to shew.

HISTORY AND DESCRIPTION OF MARGATE.

Margate lies on the ascent of a hill, on the top of which stands the church. It was formerly called St. John's, in which parish it lies; but it has changed its name since it ceased to be a little fishing town, as if it were ashamed, in its improved state, to be known by its old acquaintance.

The appellation Margate, or rather Meregate, is derived from an opening or gate, thro' which there was a small mere, or stream, running into the sea. it contains nearly 5000 inhabitants, besides the many hundreds, or rather thousands, who are brought hither by all kinds of conveyances from different parts of the kingdom, particularly from London, for the benefit of bathing:

> Whate'er from dirty Thames to Margate goes;
> However foul, immediately turns fair;
> Whatever filth offends the London nose,
> Acquires a fragrance soon from Margate air.

In fact, the fine level sandy shore at Margate, and the numerous conveniences and attractions which this place affords, both for health and pleasure, render it truly desirable.

That part of the town which originally formed the fishing village of St. John, is now called the High-street; and another detached village in the valley leading from the pier was known by the name of Lucas Dane, though both are now united by handsome ranges of buildings, many of which stand where corn was wont to grow.

The parish of St. John is about three miles and a half across each way, consisting of open corn-fields with frequent hill and dale, and containing several hamlets, and a cluster of houses, besides the town of Margate, which, in matters of civil jurisdiction, is subject to the Mayor of Dover, of which port it is an appendage; and whose chief magistrate always appoints a deputy here, but invests him with no higher power than that of a constable.*

* In 1785, Margate having risen into some consequence, an attempt was made to throw off the yoke of dependence on Dover, to accomplish which the inhabitants petitioned the crown for a charter of incorporation; but the magistrates of Dover, making a strenuous opposition, the business dropped; though it was agreed on all hands, that a better police was necessary in such a public place, and that this could only be obtained by local authorities.

The old wooden pier of Margate having become ruinous, an act of parliament was obtained in 1787, for the improvement of the town, and rebuilding and improving the pier; in consequence of which the latter has been cased on both sides with stone, and extended; but to the want of sufficient funds for farther improvements, or of aid from parliament, is very justly attributed its never having been built solid and compact enough, notwithstanding two successive attempts, to resist the force of the sea.

Margate being much exposed to the north and east has often suffered severely from tempests, and the shipping-trade, which was once considerable, is now dwindled away to a few colliers and timber ships from the Baltic, and some coasting vessels, among which the hoys or packets are the most productive, it being computed that not less than 20,000 persons annually sail to and from this port. Hence, with great truth, live stock may be regarded as the most lucrative branch of commerce in which the people of Margate are engaged.

In consequence of this profitable trade, Margate has risen from insignificance to wealth and consequence.

The increasing resort of genteel people to this place, for pleasure as well as bathing, rendered an increase of buildings necessary for their accommodation; and a new town has sprung up, to the southward of the old one, on the side of the hill near the church, while the former town has been greatly improved and enlarged.

Cecil-square, built in 1769, consists of several spacious houses, as well as commodious shops, which latter allow a view of the sea.

Hawley-square, erected in a contiguous field, is a uniform range of handsome houses.

Union-crescent, opposite to Cecil-square, is by far the most elegant and regular pile of buildings in the place. On the fort, and several other points, there are many groupes or single mansions of much beauty, commanding fine marine and land views.

To the northward of the town is a place called the Fort, which formerly had a master-gunner, and several pieces of ordnance, as a protection against privateers; but on this spot Neptune-square is now erected, and a small battery mounted on the improved construction, which equally provides for defence of, and is a real embellishment to, the town.

On the opposite hill, north-eastward of the new town, stands an assemblage of houses, called Hooper's Hill, where a curious horizontal windmill for grinding corn has been erected, at the back of the Prospect-tavern Bowling-green.

BATHING-ROOMS AND MACHINES.

The bathing-rooms are situated near the harbour, on the western side of the High-street, and though they are seven in number, and several machines belong to each, company have frequently a considerable time to wait, before they are able to procure a dip. Each person on his arrival enters his name, that he may have his regular turn, and in the mean while may amuse himself with reading the newspapers, thrumming a piano-forte, or in conversation with fellow-expectants.

The machines, which were the original invention of Benjamin Beale, a Quaker, of Margate, are on a very commodious construction, and may be driven to any requisite depth in the sea by careful guides.

There are also four marble salt-water warm baths, filled from the sea, which may be had at any temperature, on giving a short notice.

TERMS OF BATHING.

	s.	*d.*	
A lady bathing in a machine, guide included	1	3	
Two or more ladies together, guide included	1	0	each
Child in a machine, with a guide	1	3	
Two or more children together, with a guide	0	9	each
A gentleman in a machine, guide included	1	6	
Ditto, without a guide	1	0	
Two or more gentlemen, with a guide	1	3	each
Ditto, without a guide	0	9	each

Warm bath 3s. 6d. each, or seven times for a guinea.

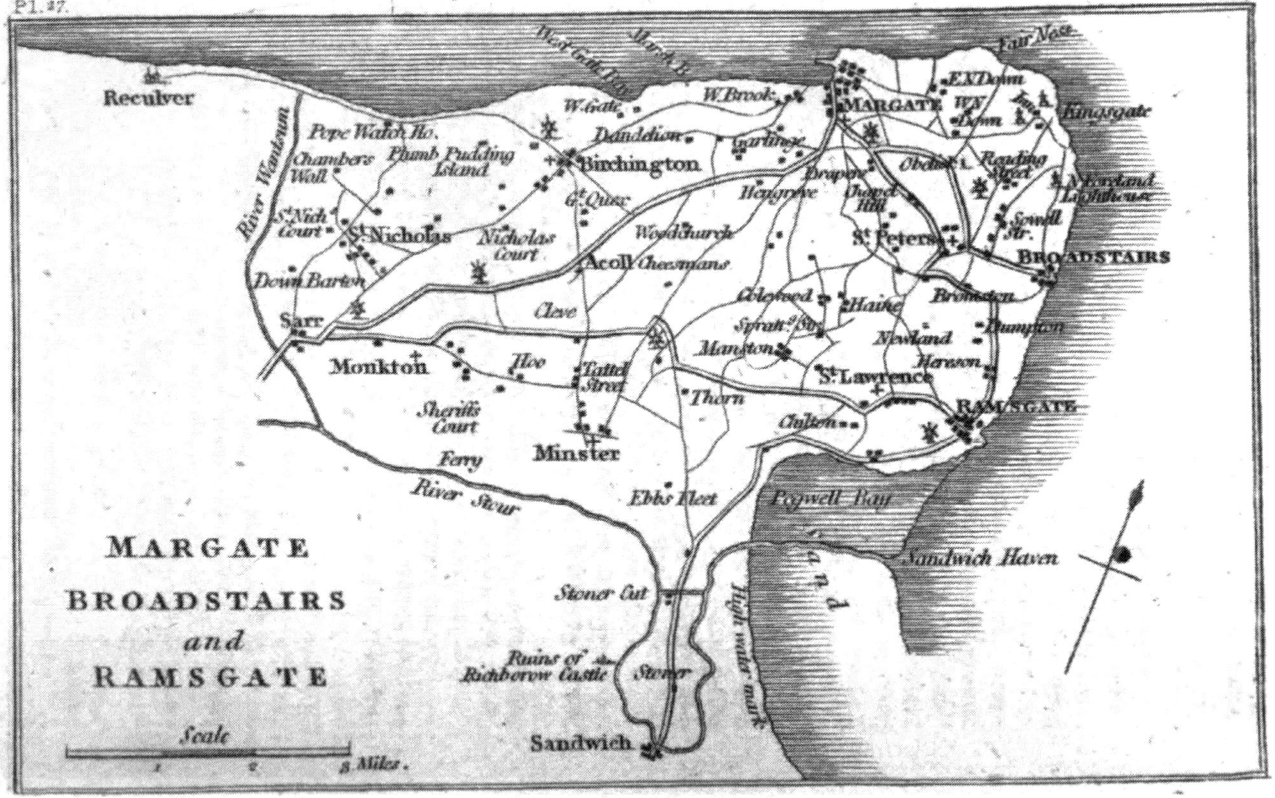
MARGATE
BROADSTAIRS
and
RAMSGATE
Scale
3 Miles.
Reculver
River Wantsum
Pope Watch Ho.
Chambers Wall
Plumb Pudding Island
St. Nicholas
Nicholas Court
Down Barton
Sarr
Monkton
Birchington
W. Gate
Dandelion
Gt. Quex
Acoll
Cheesmans
Woodchurch
Cleve
Hoo
Sheriffs Court
Ferry
River Stour
Minster
Tatted Street
Thorn
Ebbs Fleet
Stoner Cut
Ruins of Richborow Castle
Stoner
Sandwich
High water mark
Sandwich Haven
Pegwell Bay
Chilton
Manston
Coleyood
Haine
Newland
St. Lawrence
RAMSGATE
Bromston
Dumpton
W. Brook
MARGATE
Gardiner
Drapers
Hengrove
Chapel Hill
St. Peters
BROADSTAIRS
Fair Ness
E.X. Down
Kingsgate
Reading Street
North Foreland Lighthouse
Margate Road
Westgate Bay

GENERAL SEA-BATHING INFIRMARY.

In many cases cold sea-bathing is inadmissible, and in almost every case, even where it is proper, a preparatory tepid bath is to be recommended; but as warm bathing is too expensive to come within the reach of the afflicted poor, some benevolent persons, among whom was Dr. Lettsom, projected a sea-bathing infirmary, the first stone of which was laid in 1792, and it was opened in 1796, under the patronage of the Prince of Wales, and the direction of a committee.

The building, which is neat but plain, is erected at Westbrook, and is already liberally supported; but as friends to the poor and the diseased, we warmly recommend it to the continued and increasing patronage of those who have the means of rendering such a praise-worthy establishment more extensively useful.

ASSEMBLY-ROOM.

The assembly-room, situated in Cecil-square, is a splendid apartment, eighty-seven feet long, forty-three broad, and of a proportionate height. It is adorned with the busts of his present Majesty and the late Duke of Cumberland. The girandoles, mirrors, chandeliers, orchestra, and other appendages, are in the first stile of elegance. Attached are corresponding tea and card-rooms, coffee-room, and billiard-room, all belonging to the Royal Hotel, kept by Kidman, who conducts his extensive business in a manner that deserves and obtains the most distinguished patronage. The premises extend a considerable way up Cecil-street.

The season commences on the King's birth-day, and closes with the last ball-night in October. The following are the established regulations.

RULES AND ORDERS FOR ADMISSION, &c.

I. That every person, to be entitled to walk and play at cards in the rooms during the season, do subscribe 10*s.* 6*d.* and none but subscribers to be admitted into the card-room of a morning.

II. That on Mondays and Thursdays subscribers do pay 1*s.* 6*d.* admittance, and non-subscribers 4*s.* Tea at 10 o'clock, 1*s.* each.

III. That on Sundays subscribers do pay 6*d.* admittance, and non-subscribers 1*s.* Each person to pay 1*s.* for tea, if called for.

IV. That all persons playing at whist, quadrille, commerce, or loo, do pay 11*s.* for two packs of cards, and 7*s.* for a single pack. No other games to be played in the rooms, without the permission of the Master of the Ceremonies.

V. That no person be permitted to play with cards which have been left by another party.

VI. That no person be admitted into the gallery without a written order, signed by the Master of the Ceremonies; and no servants to be admitted up-stairs on any account whatever.

N. B. After 2 o'clock subscribers, or non-subscribers, to pay 6d. an hour, so long as they continue to play at cards, whether ball-night or not.

As the utmost decorum is necessary in all public assemblies, the Master of the Ceremonies requests of the company a strict compliance with the following regulations:

I. That on ball-nights no ladies be admitted into the great room in habits, nor gentlemen in swords, boots, or pantaloons; military gentlemen excepted.

II. That the balls do begin at eight o'clock, and finish at twelve precisely, even in the middle of a dance.

III. That after a lady has called a dance, when it is finished, her place in the next dance is at the bottom.

IV. That all ladies, who go down a dance, do continue in their places, till the rest have done the same.

N. B. As a deviation from this rule gives universal offence, the Master of the Ceremonies will pay the utmost attention possible, to see it strictly observed.

V. That ladies, whether of precedence or not, do take their places at the bottom, after a country-dance is begun.

VI. That the balls be on Mondays and Thursdays, and that they both be considered as undress balls. Cotillons and reels will be danced on Monday nights.

VII. That the rooms be opened on Sunday evenings for a promenade.

VIII. That two sets for country-dances be not formed 'till upwards of twenty couple stand up, to be then equally divided, and no person to change from one set to another.

IX. That no lady, &c: permit another to stand above her, after she has taken her place in a set.

☞ The Master of the Ceremonies entreats those ladies and gentlemen whom he has not the honour of knowing personally, to afford him an early opportunity of being introduced to them, as it will not only, in a certain degree, be the means of preventing improper company from coming to the rooms, but will enable him to pay every individual that attention, which it is not less his inclination than his duty to observe.

YORK HOTEL AND MARINE PARADE, &c.

The York Hotel is most delightfully situate on the Marine Parade, and commands a fine view of the harbour and the ocean. Here the accommodations are excellent, and, in addition to the comforts of an inn, there are marble warm salt-water baths, on a good construction.

For the improvement of the Marine Parade and its vicinity, a stone jetty, from the pier to the end of High-street, was completed in May, 1803. The expence was defrayed by voluntary subscription, and it is now one of the most beautiful walks that can be imagined.

There are, besides the Royal and York Hotels, various inns and taverns, where visitants may be accommodated till they have provided themselves with private lodgings, or taken up their residence in a boarding-house, the terms of which vary according to the fulness of the season, the situation, or the stile of living.

THE THEATRE-ROYAL,

Situate at the south-east corner of Hawley-square, was erected in 1787, at an expence of more than 4000*l.*; its exterior holds out but little promise, being a plain brick structure, and has more the appearance of a large barn, but the inside is fitted up in a stile of uncommon neatness and elegance; and is furnished with scenery painted by the late celebrated artist Harry Hodgings: some of them are, by connoisseurs, esteemed the chefs-d'ouvre of the art.

The próprietors are Messrs. Grub, King, Shaw, and Wells; the last gentleman is also acting-manager, and has catered with satisfaction and success för the public for many years. We always find at this Theatre sufficient talent to satisfy all but the fastidious, and the business of the scenes is well attended to. Mr. Wilmot Wells is now joint-proprietor and acting-manager of three other theatres in the vicinity of Margate, Sandwich, Deal, and Dover; and as, by this means, a yearly circuit is made out, the public has a right to expect that Margate will, in future, boast as good a company of performers as any provincial theatre in the kingdom.

LIBRARIES AND PRINTING-OFFICE.

The libraries at Margate are in the first stile of elegance, and present sufficient attractions to visit them, independent of the mental gratifications they so amply furnish, both to the scholar and to the mere reader for amusement. In particular their tables are covered with the best Magazines, Journals, and Reviews.*

* The Editor of this Work, who is also known to the public as the Author and Editor of the Picture of London, cannot forbear, as an act of justice to his readers, to insert, from that Work, a statement of indisputable Facts, relative to the scandalous and immoral abuse of criticism, which disgraces most of our Reviews These pretended criticisms are read, perhaps, with more attention by the Loungers at Watering Places than elsewhere; it is proper, therefore, that an honest guide should furnish an antidote to the dishonest practices of calumniators in the shape of anonymous critics, whose poison might have peculiar effect at a Watering Place:—

"While these professed Oracles of Literature," says the Picture of London, "spoke the language of good manners, and confined their observations to honest remarks on the Contents of the Books which they affected to notice, they deserved a qualified portion of public Confidence; but the race of Scurrility in which they have lately begun to emulate each other, and the Insults which they address to the Persons and private Characters of Authors, have rendered them at once a Disgrace to the moral Character of the country, a gross abuse of the Liberty of the Press, a Scourge of Genius, and a Nuisance to Literature.

"On ordinary occasions it would be sufficient, to refute Calumny, to state that the Author of it lurked in Concealment; but the public have been so long imposed upon by *anonymous critics*, and *anonymous criticism* has so long been received without suspicion by the unthinking, that it will be necessary to pursue these Critical Assassins to their Retreats, and to exhibit clear and correct views of the description of persons among whom they are to be found.

"We shall, in the first instance, mention as a point of fact, which no person can honestly controvert, that every one of the Reviews published, with perhaps not more than a single exception, is the Property, or in the pay of some Bookseller; and is carried on for the sole purpose of praising all his own Publications, and of *damning* and vilifying all those which he considers as interfering with his Interests.

"The pretended criticisms, which appear in these anonymous publications, *thus improperly and corruptly influenced*, are fabricated in some of the following ways, or are under the influence of some of the following abuses:

"1. *By rival Authors.*—Persons who have themselves writ-

Bettison's is situated at the north-west corner of Hawley-square; Silver's, on the north-east side of Cecil-square, opposite the Assembly-Room; and Gar-

ten on the subject treated in a new book which is to be noticed, being supposed by the conductors of Reviews to understand the point better than mere general scholars, are frequently employed to review Works in such circumstances. This is the best and perhaps the most *impartial*, judgment which an Author ever obtains; and a Critique, by a writer on the same subject, always commands, in the arrangement of a Review, a place of distinction. It need scarcely be stated, that an author seldom undertakes to write an *anonymous* critique on a *rival* publication, who, at the same time is not unprincipled enough to vent all his Envy and Malice against the book and the person of his rival; mean enough also to quote his own work with applause, and impudently contrast it with the new one. One at least of such articles appears in every Review that is published; but it generally carries with it characteristic marks of jealousy and alarm, which render it easy to be singled out by readers of ordinary discernment.

"2. *By literary Adventurers lately arrived in London, from the Provinces, or by Youths from some Scotch University.*—Young men who persuade themselves that their *great* talents can only have adequate display in the metropolis, often arrive in London; without any honest means of obtaining a livelihood, and, as a first resource, tender their service to some Bookseller who publishes a Review. Here their stock of Latin and Greek is generally placed in requisition; and, till a more honourable mode of existence presents itself, these striplings hire themselves at two or three guineas per printed sheet of 16 pages, to write opinions on all manner of subjects; and, under the mask of the important and oracular "WE," make the credulous part of the public believe them qualified to insult every man of Genius and Learning in the country.

"3. *By bankrupt Authors; the Inmates of Newgate, the Fleet, and the King's Bench.*—Half of the anonymous Criticisms which appear, are written in the Prisons of the metropolis! Some Reviews have been *solely* written and conducted by knots of imprisoned critics. No method of supporting existence in confinement is more easy and more common than the business of reviewing. It lately happened, that during several months, the Editors of two rival Reviews *chummed* together in one room in the Fleet-prison, and by their respective efforts produced two critical journals of great ner's, at the lower end of High-street, commanding a delightful marine prospect.

These libraries are well supported, and the brilli-

---

authority among the opposite partizans of Aristocracy and Democracy! The late Dr. Bisset, who, in the last years of his life had the misfortune to pass several months in the King's Bench prison, boasted to the writer of this article, and to some other friends, that he could produce two Sheets, or earn six Guineas, in a single Day, by reviewing; and that, as he had interest to obtain the insertion of different Articles relative to the same Book in various Reviews, he could rely on an income from these labours of full six guineas per week during his confinement. One of his friends, who was not before in the secret of this trade, exclaimed, " But how can you read the books, Doctor, so as to write two sheets of criticism on them in a day?"—" Read the books, man?" said the Doctor; " read them? Why, do you think a reviewer reads the books?—That shews you know nothing about the matter?" *(a)*

" 4. *By personal Friends or Enemies of the different Authors.*—The system of *anonymous* reviewing renders every Review a masked Battery, which is played according to the party of those who occupy it; either on an Author by his Enemies, or on the Public by his friends. Any Author who stoops to so wretched a Degradation, may influence in his own favour every Criticism that appears respecting his work, by Concessions, by Bribery, or by employing some known reviewer

" *(a)* If any corroboration of this point were requisite, in addition to the statement which will be found in the note in page 323, an appeal, at proper opportunities, might be made to those who have professionally a peep, in some *small* degree, behind the curtain. A Review is the constant laughing-stock in the office where it is printed. Let any journeyman printer, who has been some months employed on one, tell how many of the books noticed in it have passed through his hands, in which actually *none* of the leaves had been *cut open*, except the very passages to be copied, the table of contents, and the index; or rather (what will be infinitely less troublesome to him, and may be comprised in a very few recollections) let him tell how many were *not* in that condition. Hence the eternal complaints in Reviews, whenever a volume is published without an index, or a table of contents.

" The Reviewers are well acquainted with the remark made by Pope:

" That index learning *turns no student pale*,
But holds the eel of science by the tail." *Dunciad.*

ancy of the company who visit them is frequently such as to convert them into the appearance of assembly-rooms.

to tender his services for the occasion among the various Reviews. (b) On the contrary, any virulent Enemy of an Author may wreak his malice, by communicating *gratuitous* criticisms to the Reviewers, some of whom do not scruple to receive and insert such articles from persons wholly unknown to them; and instances have occurred, in which, with unblushing profligacy, the receipt of such anonymous criticisms has been thankfully acknowledged through the public Newspapers.

" 5. *By the Authors becoming their own Reviewers.*—It may be affirmed, without the hazard of contradiction, that in every Review that is published, there is at least one article written by the Author on his own work. As such criticisms never cost any thing, their insertion may frequently be obtained by a suitable application of the author or his friends. The proprietor himself will, under certain *circumstances*, receive these *full and able* notices; but more commonly their admission is secured by the person to whom the *examination* of the book has been assigned. The article itself values, in account with the proprietor, at a certain number of pounds, shillings, and pence; and is thought, by a hungry reviewer, to be *a good hit;* especially if accompanied by a Bank note, or an invitation to dinner. These criticisms thus written, and inserted by such means, are, without delay,

" (b) A few months ago, the writer of these remarks, who has himself played a principal part in this Farce of anonymous Criticism, was applied to on the following occasion by an old friend, a physician in the west of England, who had some time previously published a medical Work of considerable Merit and Originality. Dr. A. had, for several years, practised in a large market-town, and had secured the confidence of an extensive connection. A young physician from Edinburgh had lately settled in the same place; who, having previously passed a winter in London, had there continued his acquaintance with some young fellow-students, who from necessity had engaged themselves at three guineas per sheet to write in certain Reviews. Dr. A. at the time of finding a competitor in this stripling, was engaged on the last chapter of a work upon which he had been occupied at intervals during many years, and which was published in the following winter. The Youth, who, on account of the established reputation of Dr. A. had obtained little practice, rejoiced at the announcement of this work, as offering an opportunity by which he might avail himself of his

Warren's Printing-office, adjoining the York Hotel, is a useful establishment, and conducted by Witherden, successor to the late Mr. Warren. We re-

---

retailed again to the public in small quantities, through the advertisements in the Newspapers; and it is twenty to one but every commendatory criticism which is given at the end of a Book Advertisement in a Newspaper, has been fabricated by the Author himself, or under his immediate direction.

"6. *By Traders in Criticism.*—In London there are persons, who probably gain as much by composing separate critiques for all the Reviews on the same book, as the author who wrote it. A man of this description is generally a smatterer in some particular art or science; and when a new book appears on *his* subject, if he be not applied to by the different conductors of Reviews, he generally tenders his services, which are always accepted with thanks. Thus one and the same person assumes a dozen Identities; and by varying his language and opinions so as to meet the character, the views, and the party, of each of his employers, he praises and censures, and blows hot and cold, in the same in-

---

reviewing connection, so as to write down and depreciate the skill and science of Dr. A. He accordingly obtained from one of his friends a promise that such articles as he might send up should be inserted in several of the Reviews. Dr. A. who had for many years unsuspectingly read the Reviews as authorities not to be questioned, inspected them with particular anxiety after the appearance of his book. At length a number which contained one of the articles written by his rival, fell in his way; and the worthy physician was overwhelmed with mortification, to find himself treated as an Empiric, a Blockhead, and an Hypothesis-monger; as one whose patients, if he had any, were objects of pity, and who was himself to be pitied for the injury he had done himself and his family by such an exposure of his ignorance! It will be easier to conceive than to describe the mingled emotions of this worthy man, on finding himself so basely misrepresented; but let the reader imagine the anguish of his feelings, when one of his friends brought in a hand-bill which had the same morning been circulated through the neighbourhood, containing an extract from this very criticism, and referring to the Review published in London as the authority! He found that the Apothecary, in connection with the new physician, had been very industrious in this business; but he was too little acquainted with the arcana of *anonymous criticism*, to suspect who *might* be the author. Like an ingenuous man of letters, he printed a reply; but this only made his case the worse;

commend every visitor of Margate to call at his shop.

stant. Or perhaps a book of high price, or of considerable bulk and erudition, makes its appearance; of which, at the common price of three or four guineas per sheet, a critic who would live by his trade, could not repay himself for the cost, and for the labour of perusal, by a single criticism; he therefore accommodates various accounts of it to the passions and parties of the several Reviews; and thus the labours of the whole life of some learned and ingenious author are wholly at the mercy of this wholesale dealer in criticism; perhaps an unprincipled and malicious character, who, if known to the world, would be the last man living whose opinion would be received as an authority on this or any other subject whatever.

"7. *By contracting Critics, Master Critics, or those who review by the lump.*—Several of the Reviews, to save trouble to the proprietors and publishers, are undertaken or contracted for by one person, at so much per sheet! and this Man stands engaged either to write the entire Review himself or to get it written by others. Delegations two or three deep

---

for the dark insinuations, and the broad and course assertions of his concealed opponent, were too strong, and too operative on the minds of those who read them, to be repelled by cool argument, and by the ordinary language of a well-educated gentleman. In the mean time, a literary friend of the Doctor's, who knew something of the profligacy of criticism, convinced him that the article respecting his book was the production of some enemy; and that it would probably meet with similar treatment in some of the other reviews, if he did not exert himself to prevent it. It was therefore determined as the securest plan to avoid the mischief, that the Doctor should visit the metropolis, and through the means of his friends there, obtain introduction to the proprietors and publishers of the Reviews. The first place he drove to was the house of the narrator of these facts; and they spent two days in searching for, treating, and bribing, the hirelings who write for or superintend those journals. The result was, *that the Doctor obtained permission to send such accounts of his book as might be written by himself or his immediate friends!* The Doctor was now satisfied that the former article had been the production of some enemy; and though his soul revolted at the task he had undertaken, yet his endeavour to defeat the malice of such a wretch stimulated him to proceed. In the course of the enquiry, it appeared, that one of the new Reviews was already in possession of an article relative to the Doctor's book, and that the writer had

BOWLING-GREEN.

Attached to the Prospect Hotel, on Hooper's Hill, is a large bowling-green, with alcoves, where com-

are very common in this species of criticism. The contracting critic receives himself, perhaps, after the rate of seven guineas per sheet; but, in paying his journeyman for occasional aid, he gives but three or four guineas. The *journeyman*, too, employs commonly a species of *labourer*; whose province it is to *skim* the book, prepare the general heads of the analysis, mark the extracts, &c. &c. a business which is paid for by the job, or according to the size of the book. But many of the wholesale Critics dispense with assistance of every kind, and it is not uncommon for one or at most two, men to compile an entire Review. The writer could quote an instance which occurred a few years since, in which one Critic reviewed, in one month, no less than thirty-three books on every kind of subject.

"8. *By the profligate Calculations of the Conductors.*—It is a maxim which is constantly acted upon in the management of a Review, that it will not please all palates unless it be well seasoned: or, in the technical language of the reviewing Craft; "The Review will not sell, unless a sufficient number of authors and their books be regularly *cut up*." It becomes

treated it with great severity. This information afforded a clue for the discovery of the party; but the wary editor could not be prevailed upon to shew the manuscript, nor to promise that it should not be printed. The Doctor invited him to dinner at his hotel; treated him sumptuously; and after the bottle had been freely circulated, the article was sent for; when, after what has been stated, the reader will not be surprised at learning that the handwriting was that of the young physician who had for some time been the Doctor's insiduous rival in the country! The manuscript was confided to the Doctor, on his promising to furnish another article of equal length, gratis; and undertaking to pay for fifty of the ——— Review for three months to come, which he was to circulate and recommend in his county! On his return home, the Doctor's solicitor immediately commenced a course of legal proceedings against the young Scotchman; who, finding that he was in the Doctor's power, agreed to leave that country on their being discontinued.

pany frequently resort to drink tea; and here fireworks are occasionally exhibited.

---

therefore, part of the ordinary business of every conductor, to take care that there is no deficiency of *Sauce*, and to engage a few Miscreants who are well versed in the Language of Billingsgate. Accordingly, therefore, to the degree of honour and feeling possessed by the Conductor, or as the Review is falling or rising in Sale, it will be arranged whether the proportion of half, a third, or a quarter, of the books noticed in every number, are to be vilified! This direct ratio between the fall in sale, and scurrility of language; and between the rise in sale, and decency of language; furnishes data by which any person may, by counting the Articles of each Character, calculate at any time the Healthiness or the Decrepitude of every Review.

"9. *By the superficial View which the hired and anonymous Critic takes of the Books of which he gives an opinion.*—It is a fact which will startle some readers of these observations, but which a little attention will confirm, that the persons who write the *Monthly Catalogue* in most of the Reviews, do not *see* half the books which they characterize, but write their flippant notices solely from the advertisements in the newspapers. The present or former conductors of certain Reviews may blush to see this "secret of their prison-house" go forth to the world; but the writer pledges himself to give names and other particulars, if the fact, to the extent he has stated, should be contradicted. Let any person turn over the Monthly Catalogue of various Reviews for a few months, and he will not fail to be struck with the Imposition which has been practised on him; by observing that much above half of the silly paragraphs which are appended to the titles of pamphlets and of the other Works in this part, would apply with as much propriety to most other articles in the list, as to those to which they are assigned. This is so palpable, that no more need be urged to prove the existence of this flagrant Abuse of the name of Criticism. It may, however, be worth while to explain, that as Reviewers are paid by the Sheet, at the Rate of three, four, five, or six Guineas per 16 pages, according to their *professional* Capacity and Experience; and as the articles in the Monthly Catalogue seldom exceed a few lines each, these would not produce, on an average, more than eighteen pence or two shillings a piece, and sometimes not half of the smallest of these sums. It is absurd, therefore, to suppose, that if Reviewers mean

RELIGIOUS AND CHARITABLE ESTABLISHMENTS, &c.

The church dedicated to St. John the Baptist, stands about half a mile from the lower part of

---

to gain a livelihood, they take the trouble to read, or even to *seek* "such unproductive Trash!" *(c)* Accordingly the

"*(c)* A picture from the life will illustrate this abuse better than a multitude of observations. A principal Reviewer, possessed of more learning than prudence, had been surrendered by his Bail to the custody of the Marshal of the Fleet. From one of the Attics of that dormitory of disappointed enterprize, he addressed himself to his old Friend the Bookseller in Paternoster-row; who, knowing his talents, and fearing his resentment if neglected, sent a packet of eight or ten new publications for the nex month's Review. The critic, who always composed through the medium of an Amanuensis, caused an inquiry for one to be made in the prison; and presently a young man was enlisted in his service, who was not devoid of intelligence, but hitherto a total Stranger to the Mysteries in which he was speedily to be initiated. He seated himself with his pen in his hand; when the Reviewer untied the parcel of books; and taking up a handsome Quarto, read the title-page, and giving the volume to the Amanuensis, desired him to copy the title. While this was performing, he took several turns in the room; and having two or three times asked impatiently whether the title was finished, he ordered the Amanuensis to *write*. He then dictated an opening paragraph of considerable length; in which he abused without mercy the self-conceit of the Author in supposing himself qualified for such an undertaking, enumerated the attempts that had been made by various other Persons in the same species of writing, ascribed this Work to overweening Vanity, &c. &c. The Amanuensis was struck with surprise, for he perceived that not a leaf of the Book had been opened; and was sensible that the Dictator had not till that moment seen the Work. He was, however, staggered in this supposition, when he again heard himself commanded to *write* as follows:—"The ensuing passages alone will satisfy our readers of the justice of these conclusions; but if we chose to multiply examples of presumption and absurdity, we could fill our number with the dull conceits of this blockhead!" The Reviewer now took up the volume to seek for the passages which were to answer this prejudication, turned over its preface rapidly, and muttered, "This fellow's determined to give one all the trouble he can—No contents I

Margate. It is a large flint building, rough cast, consisting of three long low aisles, with as many chancels, separated by pillars of various forms, and

---

fact is, that this department of the Review is committed to persons kept *on the establishment*, as the manufacturing expression is; who are paid a small monthly allowance (four or five guineas) for executing it, which is divided among them, if more than one are employed, and is issued regularly

---

see!—Index perhaps?—Nor that either! Dies hard; but must be damned, for all that."—He then angrily turned over the leaves from beginning to end, read the heads of some of the chapters, and at length exclaimed, 'Yes, I have it. Write, sir. Begin, page 273, 'At the same time that,' to 278, at 'hitherto proceeded.'—Now, with the rapidity of lightning, opening the volume further on, "Write," he resumed. "This opiniated gentleman, not satisfied with differing from every writer who has preceded him, from Aristotle to Rousseau, has chosen to refute all his own doctrines by the following whimsical positions. Peace to his spirit! We hope never to wade through such another Augean stable; but long-suffering is the lot of our fraternity!"—Begin, page 417. 'With this view,' to page 420, at 'broad basis.' And again, page 432, 'It is well known,' to page 435, at 'indispensably necessary.' "We should have pitied the unfortunate publisher, who ignorantly embarked his money in this wretched performance, if the fellow had not had the impudence to fix the price of three half-guineas on a volume, which, after a patient examination, we can pledge ourselves is not worth three farthings." Thus ended the Review of a Work which has since passed through several editions; and the time spent in this fatiguing and patient investigation, was exactly twenty-five minutes.

"The Reviewer now took up the next book, which he praised as extravagantly as he had abused the other; and thus proceeded through the parcel, cutting open not more than twenty pages of the whole, and praising and damning as his Caprice, or some secret feeling, suggested, or just as it seemed to suit the humour of the moment! The time spent in thus characterizing, in dogmatical and vehement Language, two Quartos, five Octavos, two Duodecimos, and two Pamphlets, was about three hours and a half! The Amanuensis, on turning afterwards to the highly-reputed Review, in which these elaborate criticisms were displayed, found that they occupied one third of the Number! He declined any further participation in so disgraceful an employment; and has since communicated the above Facts to various persons, and among others to the writer of these remarks.

appears to have been built at different æras. At the west end of the north aisle is a square tower, crowned with a low spire, containing a peal of six bells. This

---

in weekly portions by the bookseller every Monday morning; being then frequently sent to some gaol, like the creditors' *sixpences* which become due on that day; or given to some of the upper assistants in the booksellers' shop, who are sometimes employed at this business in their spare hours.

"Such being a correct description of the persons and the practices of those who write anonymous criticisms, is it to be wondered at that these people uniformly deny their craft, and that a greater insult cannot be offered to one of these pioneers of Grub-street, than to insinuate that he writes for any Review? Not only is the practice disavowed by the whole fraternity, but if you *knew* a man to be a scribbler in Reviews, and were to ask if he wrote an article in itself meritorious, he would deem even this an insult never to be forgiven! It is true, that some Reviewers are well known: but these are generally either young in the trade, and not yet acquainted with the Infamy attached to it, or Coxcombs whose vanity supersedes every other feeling. Boys at school, and half-informed people in the country, consult these *Oracles* with so much unsuspecting credulity, that a Stripling from a Scotch University, who is admitted to perform the lowest offices in these Temples of Imposition, considers himself as having become part of the Godhead, and gives himself Airs accordingly. (*d*)

"There is, however, one class of men who give occasional countenance to Reviews, without intending the mischief which they thus assist in perpetrating. These are certain vain Pedants at our Universities, who, knowing little of the world, consider Reviews as exactly what they appear to be; and, having no readier means of displaying their knowledge of particular subjects, are often flattered by having some abstruse Work committed to them by the conductor of a Review. Tickled by this kind of compliment, they cannot conceal it from certain intimates, who circulate the fact in the University, that Dr. ——— writes for the ——— Review; and thus half the world are led to suppose that Reviews are written *con amore*, by men of real honour and

---

"(*d*) A certain Northern Review is now written chiefly in London, by young men who have but just finished attendance on their University Lectures, and the eldest of them is said not to exceed five-and-twenty years of age!

church was formerly dependent on Minster Abbey, five miles distant, but was made parochial in 1290. It contains several monuments of great antiquity,

---

learning. Professors in Universities ought to beware of thus becoming the dupes of their vanity, by enlisting themselves among a race of impostors, as base and unprincipled as ever disgraced society. Their names and their talents ought to be reserved for worthier purposes than that of giving countenance to hired and *anonymous* defamation.

"CONCLUSION. The obvious inference from all that has been stated is this: that the great vice of Reviewing exists in the *Concealment* of the Writers; and that while *anonymous* Criticism is tolerated, it is impossible even for a Conductor, who is a man of integrity, to guard against its corruption and its abuse.

"A learned and gentlemanly Critic would be able, though he signed his name to his Criticism, to perform ample justice to an author and the public. He could not adopt the impertinent, arrogant, and boasting Style of the present contemptible race of anonymous Reviewers; but his Inferences and Opinions would be received with Respect, the Public would be enlightened, and Error and Imposition would be corrected and exposed. Authors could assure themselves that their books were *seen* and *read* before they were decided upon: and the public could justly appreciate the value of a decision thus made, and thus guaranteed.

"Those who contend that Critics, under such a system, dare not do their duty, either do not understand what is meant by the word Criticism, or do not consider what was the original object of Reviews. Our essayists, from Addison to Cumberland and Knox, afford specimens of Criticism, such as no Man could have cause to disown, and such as would always be read with avidity by the public. True literary Criticism, in the hands of real Scholars, is the opposite of every thing that characterizes our modern Reviews: it never searches for personal anecdotes of an Author, or confounds, in its Disquisitions, his Foibles or Weaknesses with the Merits of his performance; it never magnifies blemishes, shuts its eye to beauties, becomes the tool of a party either political or literary, misquotes, delights in abusive and violent epithets, or arrogates its own infallibility! It is, in a word, a liberal Science, which no honest Man need be ashamed to exercise and avow; but in the hands of a CONCEALED ASSASSIN, it may be (and unfortunately is) converted to the most destructive and diabolical purposes.

and a handsome organ, presented by Mr. Cobb, senior, one of the most respectable of the inhabitants, and a banker of the place.

Seats are erected here for strangers, and on account of extra duty, the officiating clergyman has a subscription-book lying at the different libraries. This might be ordered better; a clergyman ought not to be reduced to the degradation of receiving a gratuitous subscription, like a master of the ceremonies, or the keeper of a ball-room.

In Love-lane is a meeting-house for the Baptists; and the followers of the late John Westley have a chapel in Hawley-square.

Draper's Hospital stands on a fine rising ground, and was built in 1709, by Michael Yoakley, a Quaker, who, having risen to affluence by his own industry, left this last memorial of his philanthropy. Here are nine dwellings, one of which is appropriated for an overseer, and the others for such poor men and women as are natives of the parishes of St. John, St. Peter, Birchington, and Acol. They wear a particular dress; and as their apartments are kept particularly neat, parties are frequently formed to drink tea at some of them, which answers the double purpose of charity and pleasure. In the middle of the pile is a meeting-house for the Quakers, of which sect the generality of the pensioners are.

The schools at Margate, both for young ladies and gentlemen, have gained high and deserved reputation.

MARKET, &c.

In 1777, a grant was obtained for a market on Wednesdays and Saturdays; and, in consequence of this, Margate is now well supplied with every kind of provision. An act was likewise passed, in 1787, for

True criticism, like charity, "suffereth long and is kind; envieth not; vaunteth not itself, is not puffed up; doth not behave itself unseemly; seeketh not her own; (is not selfish;) is not easily provoked; thinketh no evil: rejoiceth not in iniquity; but rejoiceth in the truth."

paving, lighting, and otherwise improving the town, and also for rebuilding the pier, as has already been noticed.

AMUSEMENTS.

Besides assemblies, plays, and libraries, walking, and riding, in fine weather, parties frequently make an excursion on the water to Deal, Dover, and other places. Some likewise take the diversion of fishing; but one amusement above all others prevails among the visitors at Margate, and that is, taking a trip to

DANDELION,

A fine rural spot, encompassed with venerable elms, about a mile and a half to the south-west of the town. Here are the remains of a mansion and fortification, which appear to have been of great strength, and are unquestionably of great antiquity, as the family of Dandelion, from which the place derives its name, became extinct in 1415, after being in possession of this seat for many ages. Numerous curiosities have been discovered here. From the heirs of the Petits, it passed to Henry Fox, Lord Holland; John Roberts, esq. was the last resident, since which it has been occupied as a place of public resort.

After Margate rose into repute as a public place, Dandelion became much frequented also; and alcoves, shrubs, flowers, a bowling-green, a platform for dancing, an orchestra, and other accommodations, are erected here for the entertainment of company, who often drink tea at this Elysian spot; and, during the season, have a public breakfast on Wednesdays, with dancing and other amusements, under the superintendance of the master of the ceremonies.

The views of the sea, of the Isle of Sheppy, and of Reculver, with its sister-spires,* are highly delightful.

* The church of Reculver was built by the Abbess of Feversham, who directed its two lofty spires to be called the Sisters, in memory of her affection for a sister, who was

SALMESTONE.

This ancient mansion, which lies between Dandelion and Draper's Hospital, formerly belonged to Christ Church, Canterbury. The lessee is bound to pay several charities; among others, a dish of pease to every poor person who claims them between May 3 and June 24, but this demand is now grown obsolete.

Hengrave, Nash-Court, Garling, Shottenden, Westbrooke, North Down, and various other places in the vicinity of Margate, deserve a visit; and company are continually passing and re-passing between this place, Ramsgate, and Broadstairs, and *vice versa*, which keeps up a constant succession of objects and scenes.

The approach to Margate was very inconvenient till of late; but some obstructions, long complained of, have been removed; and, on the whole, this public place merits the following compliment, which has been paid it.

Here music, love, and poetry combine,
Arts, wisdom, war (the wars of love) entwine.
Without the homage, which to thrones is due,
We here enjoy what they are strangers to:
Peace, health, contentment, pace these happy shores,
And lavish on us unexhausting stores.

---

wrecked here in company with her, and died a few hours after, of fear and fatigue. The Sisters are a useful sea-mark; but the encroaching waves are menacing their overthrow.

MATLOCK.

Where as proud Masson rises rude and bleak,
And with mis-shapen turrets crests the peak,
Old Matlock gapes, with marble jaws beneath,
And o'er scar'd Derwent bends his flinty teeth;
Deep in wide caves below the dangerous soil
Blue sulphurs flame, imprison'd waters boil.
Impetuous streams in spiral columns rise
Through rifted rocks, impatient for the skies;
Or, o'er bright seas of bubbling lavas blow,
As heave and toss the billowy fires below;
Condens'd on high, in wandering rills they glide,
From Masson's dome, and burst his sparry side;
Round his grey towers, and down his fringed walls;
From cliff to cliff the liquid treasure falls;
In beds of stalactite, bright ores among,
O'er corals, shells, and crystals, winds along;
Crusts the green mosses, and the tangled wood,
And sparkling plunges to its parent flood.

DARWIN'S LOVES OF THE PLANTS.

MATLOCK lies about 12 miles south-east of Buxton, and 144 from London. Its romantic beauty, as well as the salutary springs, which enrich this sequestered spot, render it dear to the man of taste, as well as to the invalid. To the former it presents Nature in her wildest and most picturesque attire; to the latter it furnishes guiety, without dissipation, and tranquillity, without gloom; while the philosopher will find a new source of gratification in those objects, which only amuse the eye of uninformed ignorance.

FEATURES OF THE ENVIRONS.

Along the course of the Derwent diversified beauty characterises every turn of the road. Rugged rocks are finely contrasted with verdure, and the trees, which cloath the slopes, lessen the impression which the sterility of the summits is apt to convey.

Near Matlock-bath the valley is bounded by two ranges of bold romantic heights, between which the

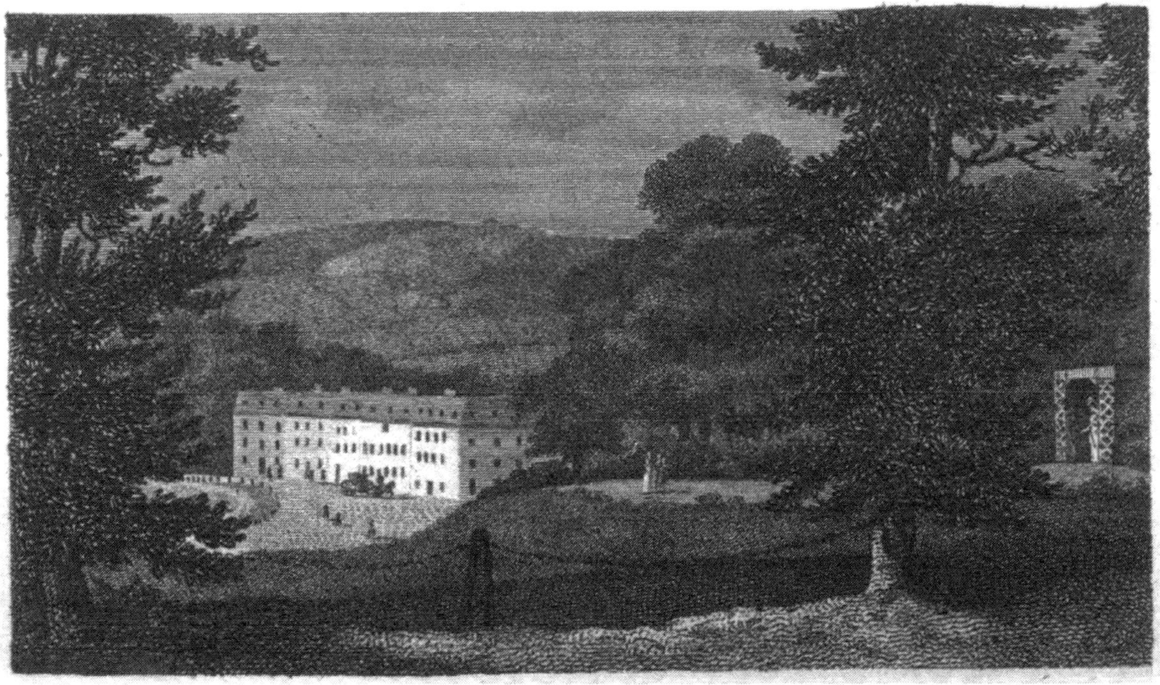

Matlock Bath from the Temple house —

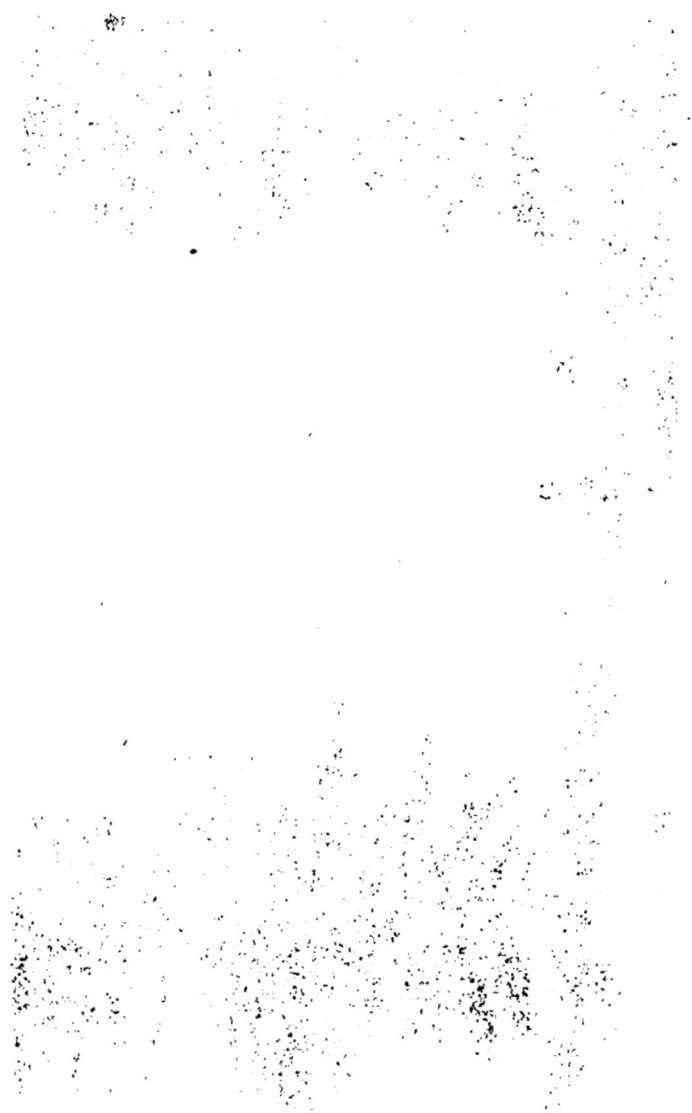

Derwent sometimes glides, in calm majesty, and sometimes dashes against opposing rocks that narrow its stream; while its banks are completely shaded with trees, and its wave is every where pellucid.

MATLOCK BATH.

The village which constitutes what is denominated Matlock-bath consists principally of three inns, known by the names of the Old Bath, the New Bath, and the Hotel, and of two commodious Lodging-houses, all situated on the south-east side of the Derwent, affording accommodation to about 400 visitors, who live here like one large family, enjoying every comfort of society without unnecessary form, and without parade, at a moderate expence.

The roads in the vicinity are as smooth as gravel-walks, and exercise either on foot, in a carriage, or horseback, is as delightful as can be conceived. It is true indeed that rain falls here more frequently and copiously than in champaign situations; but the nature of the soil quickly absorbs the superabundant moisture, and humidity is never found to affect the health of the most delicate.

The buildings at Matlock are elegantly constructed of stone, and cleanliness and comfort pervade the whole, a circumstance that has attracted the particular notice of every stranger.

The warm springs here were first noticed about 1698, when the bath was paved and built by the Rev. Mr. Fern, of Matlock, and Mr. Heyward, of Cranford. It afterwards fell into the hands of Mr. Wragg, who, to confirm his title, took a lease of it from the different lords of the manor for 99 years; and, thus secured, he built a few small rooms adjoining to the bath for the accommodation of company.

Two gentlemen of Nottingham having purchased the lease and property of Mr. Wragg, erected several accommodations on a large scale, and made a road, by which a communication was opened with the southern parts of Derbyshire.

Some years afterwards another spring was discovered, at the distance of about a quarter of a mile from the old one; and here likewise a bath, and other appendages, were erected.

At a still later period, a third spring was found, between 3 and 400 yards to the eastward of the original bath; and this being likewise enclosed, and a lodging-house built, by gradual enlargements the latter has risen to a considerable degree of elegance, and now forms a very commodious hotel.

The fame of Matlock water seems to have regularly encreased, and the number of visitors has been proportionably augmented. It has been analysed by several eminent physicians, who agree that it is grateful to the palate, though they differ somewhat on its component parts. A gallon of it has been found to contain 40 grains of sediment, which seems to consist of nitre, alkaline earth, and marine salt. It appears to have a strong resemblance, in its qualities and effects, to Bristol water; but, from its being unimpregnated with any mineral spirit, appears less likely to accelerate the pulse, and therefore may be used more freely.

Various theories have been formed respecting the cause of its heat, which is about 68 degrees. Dr. Darwin, with whose beautiful verses on the subject we have enlivened this article, thinks that it originates in the steam raised from deep subterraneous fires, and not from the decomposition of pyrites, more superficially situated. A late writer on the subject, Mr. Lipscomb, from the reflection that a portion of saline matter has been dissolved in these waters, which, it is well known, will dissolve lime in considerable quantities, conjectures, and apparently on good grounds, that the water of these springs, being previously impregnated salt, becomes saturated with lime in its passage, and is afterwards decomposed by the addition of pyrites dissolved in the rain water, which percolates through the super-incumbent strata.

VIRTUES OF MATLOCK WATERS.

Matlock waters have been recommended in glandular affections, rheumatism, and consequent debility, in the early periods of consumption, gravel, scrophula, calculous complaints, cachexy, gout, diabetes, obstructions, biliary concretions, and disease in general arising from relaxation. In all such cases they have been used with manifest advantage, when recourse has been had to them in time; but, it is to be lamented, that mineral waters in general are seldom resorted to, till medical aid has failed, and the patient is almost hopeless.

The usual times of bathing, and drinking the waters, is before breakfast, or between breakfast and dinner, and the Matlock season commences with April, and ends with October.

Those who drink the waters should begin with a small quantity at first, and encrease it gradually, according as their stomachs may be found to bear it. In this, however, they should be guided by the advice of the physician, and the nature of their disorder.

The votive crutch hung up here by numbers, who have tasted the efficacy of the Matlock waters, is a convincing trophy of their virtues; and the experience of a century, with the feelings of those who annually resort to this place, testify the numerous cures that they have performed.

MISCELLANEOUS INFORMATION.

In such a sequestered spot, amusements cannot be expected to be much diversified, but what the place admits of are innocent and cheap. Besides the Bowling-green, each of the inns has a billiard-table. Balls are occasionally held here; but it depends on the pleasure of the company when, and a regular master of the ceremonies, it is probable, will never be required here.

Provisions of all kinds are plentifully supplied from the neighbouring markets; and board and lodging may generally be obtained on moderate terms.

Each of the inns furnishes excellent post-chaises; and open-carriages and saddle-horses may generally be hired, for which the goodness of the roads, and the many agreeable rides in the vicinity, offer a frequent inducement.

The post comes in every morning at six o'clock, and goes out at the same hour in the evening.

THE VILLAGE OF MATLOCK.

This village lies about a mile and a half from Matlock Bath, on the banks of the Derwent, over which there is a neat stone bridge. It is chiefly inhabited by persons engaged in the lead mines, and in the cotton manufactories.

Matlock, from the time of Edward I. to the 4th of Charles I. continued a portion of the duchy of Lancaster, but is now divided into several small shares. The population of the whole parish amounts to about 2350 persons. The church is a rectory, in the patronage of the Dean of Lincoln. It is small and unadorned, and destitute of any curious monuments; but the living is reckoned worth 300*l.* a-year.

About a mile from the village stands what is called the Boat-house, built on the base of a rock. It has a good garden, and an assembly-room.

THE DERWENT, AND ITS SCENERY.

The Derwent rises in the northern extremity of Derbyshire, and, after a winding course through a hilly country, falls into the Trent, a few miles beyond Derby. It is said to be warmer than the generality of rivers, which probably arises from its flowing over beds of limestone. Certain it is, that, in the severest winters, it is less frozen than the Trent, and sooner open.

It produces trout and grayling in abundance, and affords the company at Matlock the diversion of angling in great perfection.

The scenery on its banks is highly interesting. From the turnpike-gate at Matlock to the Old Bath, the margin is one complete incrustation of tophus, which gradually acquires such a degree of hardness that most of the buildings in the vicinity are built with it.

The cliff, which bounds the eastern bank, particularly that part of it called the High Torr, is remarkably bold and picturesque. The prospect of the cliff from the old Bath is also very striking; and that from the front of Froggatt's Hotel, though not the most wild and romantic, is the most pleasing to the eye. The trees, which cloath the opposite steep, exhibit a beautiful variety of tints, which finely contrast with the bare and rugged protuberances of the rock that advance to meet the view.

The Derwent, murmuring along, forms a gentle curve in front of the Hotel, and the ground here is laid out with abundant taste and adaptation, though nature prevails, as if disdaining the controul of art.

WALKS AND RIDES ROUND MATLOCK.

The entrance into Matlock Dale is through a blasted rock, opened on purpose, and the effect of which is very striking. On the left hand of the Dale are prodigiously high and barren rocks, and on the other hand they form almost a perpendicular rampart of two or three hundred feet, partially shaded by trees and shrubs, which soften the general awfulness of the scene. The lower part of the Dale is well wooded, and the projecting rocks are mixed with luxuriant foliage, which likewise overhangs the river during a course of two miles.

Crossing the Derwent in a boat above the Old Bath, will display the sublime features of the Dale to the best advantage. On landing, three walks are seen pointing through the wood in as many ifferent directions. Two of them, by an ascending labyrinthine path along the side of the Dale, reach the summit of the cliff, and thus give a new and different view of the scenes already observed. The other path, called the Lover's Walk, runs along the side of the river through over-arching trees, which have been cut to allow a passage.

Besides these, there is another very pleasant walk through a grove, lying between the old and new bath.

CROMFORD-MILL.

The cotton manufactory established at Cromford, on the banks of the Derwent, in this vicinity, will claim the notice of every stranger. This was the first mill erected by Sir Richard Arkwright, whose mechanical skill was equally honourable and advantageous to himself and to his country. The machinery must be seen; for no words can give a clear idea of it; and justly may we say with Mr. Pilkington, in his view of Derbyshire, "that every distinct part is sufficient to excite admiration, and nothing less than an unbounded invention could have combined together, in one machine, so great a variety of original movements."

The inventor of this machinery, which equally lessens labour, and saves time, was originally a barber, and he had difficulties to contend with, which a common man would have sunk under. Fortunately he met with friends capable of appreciating his merit, and he lived to surmount all opposition, and to enjoy the rewards of his genius. Besides this, which lies between Cromford and Matlock Bath, here are two other cotton-mills, on the same construction.

WELLERSLEY.

When Sir Richard Arkwright had established a cotton-mill here, he naturally wished to erect a mansion for himself, and he chose a delightful spot near the extremity of Matlock Dale.

The house is built of white stone, and commands a very interesting landscape, which must have been endeared to the heart of the late possessor by the reflection, that under his auspices the whole district was enriched, and comfort and plenty introduced where they had hitherto been strangers. The Derwent washes the foot of the knoll on which the house stands, and the opposite side of the vale is a continuous range of rocky cliffs, interspersed with bushes, while the eminences are capped with firs.

The gardens are entered by a neat lodge. Formerly they were open to the company at Matlock, but in consequence of some irregularities, they are now only shewn by a guide, twice a week. The house has several neat rather than elegant apartments; but the appendages are in the first style of magnificence.

Between the river and the cliff is a small chapel, elegantly built of hewn stone, erected and endowed by Sir Richard, with a rent-charge of 50*l.* a-year, and by an augmentation with Queen Anne's bounty, the cure is now worth 70*l.*

From an eminence called Wild Cat Torr, on the summit of the rock on the eastern side of the Derwent, is a fine bird's-eye view of Matlock and the neighbouring cliffs—of the road to Wirksworth—of the Heights of Abraham, a beautiful eminence planted with fir-trees—of Arkwright's cotton manufactory—and of Saxten's bowling-green, with various inferior objects.

PETRIFYING SPRING.

Near the western bank of the Derwent, which has already been noticed as a complete mass of tophus, rises a petrifying spring, into which whatever is thrown speedily becomes incrusted, and at length wholly petrified. Among the curiosities which the keeper of this spring shews in his collection, are an old wig and a hair broom, which evince the wonderful powers of this water.

CAVERNS, AND SPAR ORNAMENTS.

It is impossible to enumerate half the wonders of nature which Matlock and its vicinity produce, and therefore we must confine ourselves, in a great measure, to the works of art, with an intermixture of some which no art can furnish.

Cumberland Cavern, which is generally visited, is said to have formerly communicated with the entrance of an old lead mine, and, therefore, is a mixed production; but Smedley's Cavern is only the sport of nature, though it was inaccessible till the person, whose name it bears, after seventeen years labour and perseverance, opened a communication with it, and he now acts as a guide to display its beauties. Here he found immense treasures of spar, and other curious minerals and fossils, with which his museum, opposite the new bath, is always plentifully stored.

The person who shews the Cumberland cavern has likewise a repository of the same kind near Froggatt's hotel, and visitors to Matlock constantly purchase some of those beautiful stalactite ornaments, which are manufactured and sold here.

It is wonderful to behold what elegant curiosities are formed from spars and petrifactions. Smedley has followed this business for more than thirty years; and, though it is doubtful whether he was the original inventor, he has certainly carried the art to the highest pitch of perfection. Vases, urns, pedestals, pyramids, ink-stands, chimney ornaments, salts, and various other articles, exquisitely shaped and polished, may always be procured in his repository.

KEDDLESTON, &c.

Fourteen miles from Matlock, is Keddleston, the elegant seat of Lord Scarsdale, an object of universal admiration. This elegant mansion, equally an honour to the country and to the nobleman who reared it, stands in a spacious park, well stocked with deer, and adorned with venerable oaks. The north front, measuring 360 feet in length, consists of a centre and two pavilions, connected with it by corridors. The portico is supported by beautiful Corinthian columns; the hall is a most magnificent apartment; and almost every room is embellished with the choicest works of art. The paintings and statues are far too numerous to be particularized.

At the verge of Keddleston-park, an inn has been erected by Lord Scarsdale, for the accommodation of company resorting to the mineral springs in the vicinity. These are of the sulphureous kind, and very much resemble the water at Harrowgate in their qualities and effects.

At Quarndon, about a mile from Keddleston, is a chalybeate spring, which is much frequented in summer. It appears to be strongly tonic.

ASHBORNE.

Ashborne is a pleasant town, standing on the side of a hill. It is built of brick, and commands many picturesque views over this romantic country. In the church is a singularly beautiful monument, erected by Sir Brooke Boothby, to the memory of his only daughter, a child of six years of age. No person who passes this way should overlook it. Simplicity and elegance appear in the workmanship; tenderness and innocence in the image. In short, it is one of the most interesting and pathetic objects of the kind in England; and the different inscriptions in Latin, Italian, French, and English, are in perfect unison with the sculpture. Beneath, on the pedestal, appears—

To Penelope,
Only Child of Sir Brook and Dame Susannah Boothby,
Born April 11th, 1785, died March 13th, 1791.
She was in form and intellect most exquisite. The unfortunate Parents ventured their all in this frail Bark,
and the wreck was total.

OKEOVER.

Okeover, the seat of a gentleman of the same name, contains a collection of paintings by the first masters. A holy Family, by Raphael, is reckoned the finest production of that great artist.

DOVEDALE, &c.

At Ashborne it is usual to take a guide, to visit the romantic and sublime beauties of Dovedale, so named from the river Dove winding through it. Not far within the Dale, is the frightful eminence from whence the Rev. Mr. Langton, dean of Clogher, who rashly attempted to ascend it on horseback, with a young lady behind him, was precipitated, and killed. His companion, a Miss La Roche, escaped destruction, being caught in her descent by the hair in a bramble-bush. The horse likewise was saved.

Proceeding onwards, arrive at a grand arch in a rock, called Reynard's Hole; beyond which is Reynard's Hall and Kitchen. This station affords a beautiful and spacious view of the Dale, with its rocks and pendent woods.

Middleton Dale, Monsel Dale, and Eyam Dale, also respectively possess their appropriate beauties.

Near the village of Whetton, a mile or two above Dovedale, is a spacious cavern, about the middle of the ascent of the mountain, called Thor's House; and below is an extensive and romantic common, where the rivers Hamps and Manifold sink into the earth, and rise again in Ilam Gardens, the seat of John Port, esq. about three miles below. The Druids are said to have offered human sacrifices to Thor, inclosed in wicker-idols; a circumstance on which Dr. Darwin, while he paints the local scenery, most poetically enlarges.

Where Hamps and Manifold, their cliffs among,
Each in his flinty channel winds along,
With lucid lines the dusky moor divides,
Hurrying to intermix their sister tides.
Where still their silver-bosom'd nymphs abhor
The blood-smear'd mansion of gigantic Thor—
Erst fires volcanic in the marble womb
Of cloud-wrapp'd Whetton rais'd the massy dome;
Rocks rear'd on rocks, in huge disjointed piles,
From the tall turrets, and the lengthen'd aisles;
Broad pond'rous piers sustain the roof, and wide
Branch the vast rainbow ribs from side to side.
While from the above descends, in milky streams,
One scanty pencil of illusive beams,

Suspended crags, and gaping gulfs illumes,
And gilds the horrors of the deepen'd glooms,
—Here oft the Naiads, as they chance to stray,
Near the dread Fane, on Thor's returning day,
Saw from red altars streams of guiltless blood,
Stain their green reed-beds, and pollute their flood;
Heard dying babes in wicker prisons wail,
And shrieks of matrons thrill th' affrighted gale;
While from dark caves infernal echoes mock,
And fiends triumphant shout from ev'ry rock!

HADDEN HALL.

Near the town of Bakewell stands Hadden Hall, an ancient mansion, belonging to the Duke of Rutland, which is still venerable in its ruins. Passing through the massive portal, and the first quadrangle, enter the Hall, guarded by the branching antler, the pride of ancient nobility, and the dread of modern. The rooms are still hung with tattered tapestry, rusty helmets, corselets, and breast-plates, which give them a more desolated appearance. In some places, painted glass defies the access of light, and naked walls exclude every idea of cheerfulness.

CHATSWORTH, THE SEAT OF THE DUKE OF DEVONSHIRE.

This magnificent seat, which is esteemed one of the wonders of the Peak, stands at the easy distance of twelve miles from Matlock, and is commonly visited by such as make any stay at the baths. It is impossible to say which is most deserving of admiration, the grandeur of the building, or the wild romantic country in which it is situated.

The position of Chatsworth-house is no less striking than the pile itself. It stands in a spacious and deep valley, near the foot of a lofty mountain, covered with wood. The Derwent winds before it, over which an elegant bridge is thrown. The architectural beauties of this place are too various to enumerate. The rooms are fitted up in a princely stile, and adorned with the finest productions of art. Here the unfortunate Mary Queen of Scots was confined sixteen years, and here Marshal Tallard was sent, after the battle of Blenheim.

The extent of the south-front of Chatsworth is 182 feet, and that of the west 180. The window-frames on the south are entirely gilt; and the splendour of the interior forms a striking contrast with the natural scenery of the environs. It has been the seat of the noble family of Cavendish for two centuries. On the pediment of the south-front is inscribed the family motto—CAVENDO TUTUS.

The gardens, though laid out in the ancient stile, still attract notice on account of their singular and fantastic decorations. We describe them in the words of Mr. Lipscomb. "The great cascade descends with considerable noise and impetuosity, by a flight of stone steps, down a steep hill, for 2 or 300 yards, and then sinks in the earth, and disappears. At the head of this cascade is a temple, sheltered by a venerable wood.

"In the front of the building, over the entrance, the figure of Nilus reclines on an urn, from which a stream of water descends, as also from a dragon, on each side of the cornice, from the mouths of lions, or perhaps sea-monsters, and from the urns of two sea-nymphs into a bason, in which the water also arises in the shape of two fine spreading trees or fans. When the bason is filled, the cascade begins to play.

"There is also a copper tree, the branches of which produce an artificial shower; but these conceits are rather curious than useful. A *jet d'eau*, however, must be excepted, which, throwing up a strong column of water, to the height of ninety feet, has a striking effect.

"The sea-horses, in a circular bason, near the south front of the house, are both clumsy and puerile.

"These works are supplied by a reservoir, which is said to cover sixteen acres of ground."

Other objects of attraction, in the vicinity of Matlock, are the silk mills at Derby; the lead mines near Wirksworth; the rocking-stone, or Druidical altar, on a hill, called the Riber, and the seat of Mr. Gell, at Hopton.

Many curious objects are also common to the visitors of Buxton and Matlock; and to the description of the former place we beg leave to refer them.

The botanist, the mineralogist, and the fossilogist, will all find gratification in examining the copious stores in each class of nature, within the precincts of the Peak.

RAMSGATE.

The Isle of Thanet, small and circumscribed as its limits are, contains no fewer than three sea-bathing places, Margate, Ramsgate, and Broadstairs, which are here arranged in the rank of celebrity they respectively hold.

Ramsgate, a hamlet belonging to the parish of St. Lawrence, is situate about five miles to the south of Margate, in a valley opening to the south-east, and commands a delightful prospect of the British channel.

Anciently it was a poor fishing town, containing a few mean houses; but about somewhat more than a century ago, its inhabitants participating largely in the trade to Russia and the east country, it began to emerge from its original insignificance; and since it became known and frequented as a bathing-place, the old houses have not only been improved, but many new and handsome buildings have been erected, particularly in Albion-place, Chapel-place, Prospect-row, Nelson's Crescent, and on Sion-hill. In short, a spacious new street, and many large and elegant detached edifices, have sprung up here within a few years, for the accommodation of summer visitors. But though it may be considered as the rival of Margate, and certainly is filled with very respectable, and even more select company, it is never likely to supplant that favourite place; especially as the point of land between them, the North Foreland, is sometimes weathered with difficulty, and, in consequence, three-fourths of the people who visit Margate coming by the hoy, are induced to stop where the voyage ends. It should be noticed, however, that Ramsgate has its hoy as well as Margate; but it is much less crowded with live stock; and the place itself wants many of those attractions which draw the young and the gay to its neighbour, particularly a theatre.

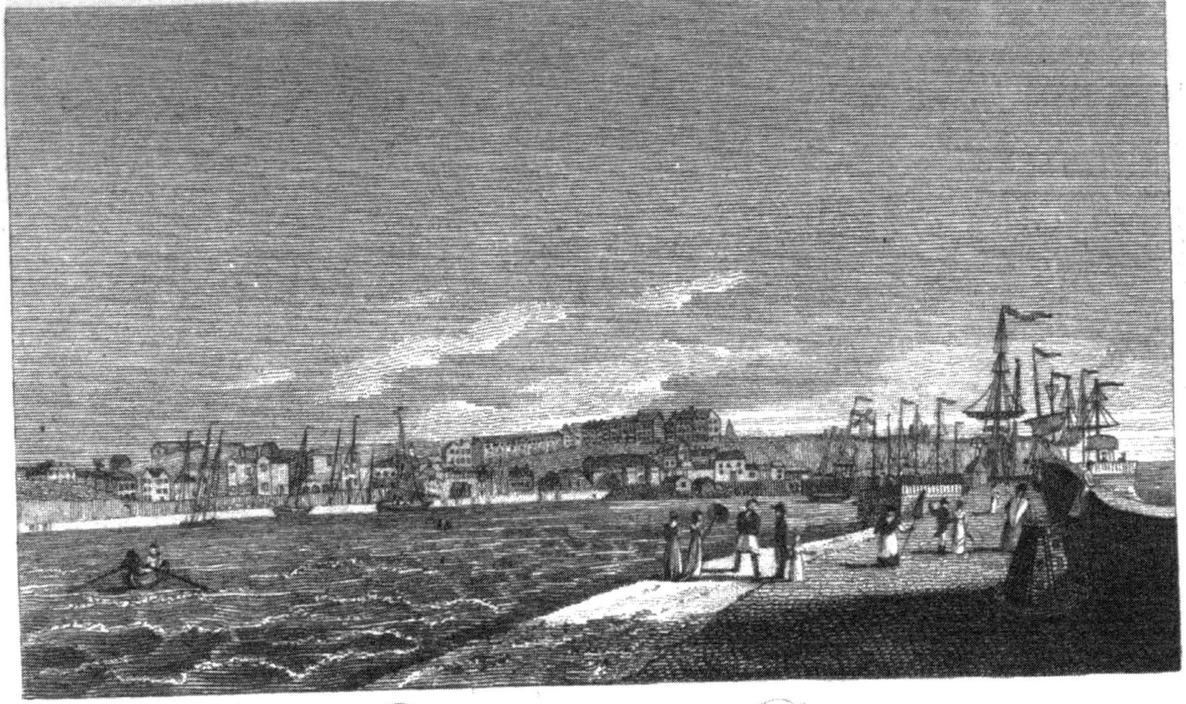

Ramsgate, from the Pier.

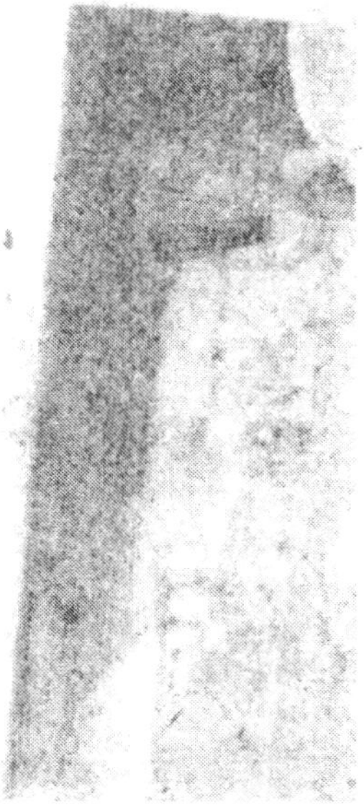

Ramsgate lies within the liberty of the cinque-ports, being an ancient appendage to Sandwich, the mayor of which appoints his deputy or constable here.

THE PIER.

The pier of Ramsgate is one of the most magnificent structures in the kingdom, and the greatest beauty of the place. It is built of Portland and Purbeck stone, at the expence of some hundred thousand pounds.

This great work was begun in 1749; it extends about 800 feet into the sea before it forms an angle, and is twenty-six feet broad at the top, including the parapet. The south-front is a polygon, its angles five on a side, each 450 feet, with octagons of sixty feet at the ends, and the entrance 200 feet. The harbour contains an area of forty-six acres, which after this great work was finished, according to the first design, becoming choaked up with mud, for want of a back water, the celebrated engineer, Mr. Smeaton, was called in, who, by erecting a cross-wall in the uppermost part of the harbour, filled with sluices, and extending the pier 400 feet from the extremity of the last head, effected all that was wanted, and facilitated the entrance of ships in hard gales of wind; for whose reception and safety on this exposed coast the whole was originally undertaken.

A dry dock has also been formed, and store-houses erected for every necessary purpose.

In addition to these improvements, within the last ten years, a new stone light-house has been built on the west head, furnished with Argand lamps and reflectors, a handsome house for the trustees to transact business when at Ramsgate, and another for the residence of the harbour-master, a watch-house, and other appropriate appendages to this immense national work: and it is said, that the trustees have it farther in contemplation to form a spacious wet-dock.

This harbour, though originally intended for ships of 800 tons burthen and under, has been so much improved, that it is now capable of receiving vessels of 500 tons. During a dreadful gale, in 1791, upwards of 130 sail took shelter here, and since that time 300 ships at once have sought this asylum.

GRAND PROMENADE.

When we have mentioned the vast length and breadth of the pier, it is almost unnecessary to observe, that it forms the favourite walk for company; and certainly none can be more delightful, or more salubrious. It commands views of the Downs, the coast of France, the towns of Deal and Sandwich, and many of the hills and fertile vallies of East Kent, while the sea-breezes can be equally enjoyed here, as if a person were floating on the bosom of the deep.

BATHING-PLACE, &c.

The bathing-place lies in front of a long line of high chalky rocks at the back of the pier, and is composed of a reddish sand, soft and pleasant to the feet. Machines ply here in the same manner as at Margate, though they are not so numerous. The rooms for the accommodation of bathers are commodious; and Dyason, of the bath-house, has erected four warm salt-water baths, also a plunging and shower-bath, to which are attached convenient waiting and dressing-rooms. This ingenious and useful undertaking deserves every encouragement.

ASSEMBLY-ROOM.

The assembly-room is situate near the harbour, and is a neat fabric, with annexed coffee, tea, billiard and card-rooms. The amusements are under the direction of the master of the ceremonies of Margate.

The assembly-room, formerly kept by Mr. Heritage, is now conducted by Mr. Goodyer; and Mrs. Sackett is succeeded in the tavern by Mr. Page, of the London Hotel, which is likewise an excellent house of accommodation. There are several other inns and public-houses for the reception of travellers and visitors; and lodging and boarding-houses suited to all conditions.

LIBRARIES.

Burgess's library, in the High-street, is valuable and extensive, and has a good stationary and toy-shop attached to it.

There is another spacious and elegant library in Cliff-street, Sion-hill, kept by Mrs. Witherden.

MISCELLANEOUS PARTICULARS RELATIVE TO RAMSGATE.

In the reign of Queen Elizabeth, it appears that there were only twenty-five inhabited houses in this place, and a proportionable number of inhabitants. About twenty years ago, the population amounted to 1810; and in 1801 the return made to parliament was 3,300, a most astonishing increase, and the best proof of the rapidly rising prosperity of the town.

Ramsgate has no theatre, which, from its vicinity to Margate, is probably little wanted.

In 1785, a handsome chapel was built here, which was consecrated by the Archbishop of Canterbury, in 1795. The Independents and Baptists have also their respective meeting-houses.

The town is well paved, lighted, and watched; and a market has been established, which is well supplied, under the authority of parliament, which likewise passed an act in 1786, for establishing a court of requests in Ramsgate and its environs, for the recovery of small debts.

Several respectable seminaries, for the education of young ladies and gentlemen, have been established here.

RIDES AND WALKS ROUND RAMSGATE.

Many objects and situations being equally common to the visitors of Margate, Ramsgate, and Broadstairs, we refer our readers to the first and last, for what may seem deficient here.

East Cliff Lodge, about half a mile from Ramsgate, is an elegant gothic villa, enjoying the most picturesque views.

Ellington, about half a mile to the west of Ramsgate, was long the seat of a family of the same name. It afterwards came to the Spracklyns, one of whom having murdered his wife, was tried at Sandwich,* and executed for the same. It is now the property and residence of John Garrett, esq.

Pegwell, about a mile to the west of Ramsgate, is seated on a spacious bay of the same name, where the inhabitants catch various kinds of shell and flat fish, &c. Belle Vuë, an inn intended for the reception of parties of pleasure from the neighbouring towns, is most agreeably situated. Attached to it are pleasure-gardens, and alcoves for summer-visitors. This pleasant spot, however, as well as other places of public resort, at many of the sea-bathing-places, is rendered disgusting by the nauseating smell and appearance of the remains of millions of marine insects, of the crab-kind, which are devoured by visitors, who do not seem to reflect, that for the gratification of a wanton appetite, these curious and harmless animals are boiled alive!

The villa of Counsellor Garrow, and Belmont, the seat of Thomas Warre, esq. stand in this vicinity.

St. Lawrence, in which parish Ramsgate lies, is a pretty village, situated on a hill, commanding many extensive prospects. The church is very ancient, and the tower, in particular, is of curious Saxon architecture.

Manston, a village about a mile and a half from St. Lawrence, enjoys a fine romantic situation, and forms an agreeable walk either from Margate or Ramsgate. Here are chalk-pits formed something like the aisles of a gothic cathedral, by the whim of

* The place of trial and subsequent condemnation deserves to be particularly mentioned, as no other instance is recorded of the like jurisdiction being exercised at Sandwich.

a person of the name of Troward, who formerly lived here. These have been considered by "would-be antiquaries," as ancient places of refuge during the incursions of the Danes.

The chapel belonging to Manston Court, is a picturesque ruin, over-run with ivy.

Birchington is a large village, about four miles west from Margate, standing half a mile from the sea-shore. The church is a handsome pile, and contains many ancient monuments of the families of Quex and Crispe. At the mansion of a gentleman, of the name of Quex, near this place, William III. used to reside, till the wind favoured his passage to Holland, and his bed-room is still indicated.

The healthiness of this village is evinced by the longevity of its inhabitants, numbers of whom live to be between eighty and one hundred.

St. Nicholas, another beautiful village, lies about two miles to the westward of Birchington. The church stands on a rising ground, and has three beautiful Saxon arches.

Saare, now a small village at the western extremity of the island, was once a place of some repute. Being half-way between the principal towns of Thanet and Canterbury, it has still two good inns of accommodation.

Two miles to the eastward of Saare stands the village of Monkton, so called from having been the property of the monks. The church is ancient; in the chancel are twelve stalls, and in the windows the portraits of several priors on painted glass. At the west end, are these monkish lines in black letter:

Insula rotunda Tanatos, quam circuit unda,
Fertilis et munda, nulli est in orbe secunda.

Thanet's round isle, compass'd with water round,
Fruitful and neat; the like's not to be found.

About two miles from this place is the ancient town of Minster, where Domneva, daughter of Ercembert, King of Kent, founded an abbey, in 670, and herself became the first abbess. Her daughter Mildred succeeded her, and became so eminent for piety, that the convent was called by her name, and she was canonized.

The church of Minster is the most ancient structure in the island; it has three aisles, and eighteen collegiate stalls in the choir. On the floor are several ancient flat grave-stones, probably the memorials of some of the religious belonging to the house.

The remains of ancient Stonar, supposed to have been the *Lapis Tituli* of the Romans, stand near Sandwich, in the road from Ramsgate. In the time of the Conqueror, it appears to have been a large and populous place, but being plundered and burnt by the French, in 1385, it never recovered the misfortune. Some valuable salt-works have been erected here.

Richborough, the Rutupiæ of the Romans, lies a mile to the right of Stonar. Here the Roman forces generally landed, and many of their coins are still found near the spot. It continued to be a place of importance for nearly a thousand years, but was finally ruined by the Danes, about 1010. Some remains of its castle are still to be seen, overgrown with ivy, and part has tumbled into the deep. Dr. Battely, in his *Antiquitates Rutupinæ*, gives an interesting account of this place.

Mount Pleasant, a house of entertainment, to which parties of pleasure resort, stands on an eminence, about half a mile north-west of Minster, and is universally admired for the beauty of its prospects, which take in the whole of Thanet, Reculver, the ancient Regulbium, the Isle of Shepey, the Nore, the coast of Essex, the British Channel, the cliffs of Calais, and many other places.

At Reculver, which is much visited, are some remains of a fort, said to have been built by Severus, about 235, and many Roman coins and other antiquities belonging to that nation are still occasionally discovered here. It is now, however, more remarkable for its church, or rather for its two spires, called the Sisters, the origin of which has already been mentioned. Here the Saxon kings had a palace, and the body of Ethelbert is said to have been buried in the church of Reculver.

The sea having made such inroads at this place, and washed away part of the church-yard, with the remains of those deposited there, it is considered necessary to take down this ancient building and sea-mark, and to erect a smaller one near the said spot. The lead from the roof is already taken off, in consequence of such determination.

REDCAR.

This charming sea-bathing place is situated in the North-riding of the county of York, and in that part of it called Cleveland.

Redcar is 252 miles from London, 56 from York, and 47 from Scarborough.

The air of this part of the county is most salubrious, and provisions of every description are in great abundance, and to be obtained at a moderate price. Shell, aud every other kind of fish, is in the greatest plenty, being daily caught, by fishermen belonging to the place, in considerable quantities. There is a post every day, except Sunday and Tuesday, from hence to Gainsborough (the post town), which leaves Redcar by a little before seven in the morning, and returns about one o'clock in the afternoon.

The bathing is excellent: and the sands are certainly not inferior to any in the kingdom, being perfectly hard and dry for an extent of nearly eight miles, and their very gradual declivity equally adapts them for the promenade or the carriage. There are also many beautiful drives in the vales of Cleveland, surrounding Redcar (and upon good roads), which for a distance of several miles may be taken in any direction, without being impeded by a turnpike-gate.

There are two Inns, for the accommodation of any part of the company who may chuse to reside at them, both of which have daily ordinaries.

The remains of the Abbey at Gainsborough is an object particularly worthy of observation.

The seats in the neighbourhood are Lord Dundas, at Upleathorn; Hon. Laurence Dundas, at Marske; Sir Charles Turner's, at Kirkleathorn; Robert Challoner, esq. near Gainsborough; John Wharton, esq. at Skelton Castle.

The direct road from London is by the great north road, to Thirsk, in Yorkshire:

	Miles.
From Thirsk, to the Cleveland Inn	10
—— Cleveland Inn to Stokesley	8
—— Stokesley to Redcar	15

The direct road from Scarborough.

Scarborough to Whitby	21
Whitby to Gainsborough	21
Gainsborough to Redcar	5

COATHAM

Is about a quarter of a mile to the west of Redcar, contains two Inns for the reception of the company, and from its proximity, varies but little in its sands, drives, &c. &c. from what has been said in the description of the foregoing place

SCARBOROUGH.

The double attraction of sea-bathing and mineral waters, which this place possesses, renders it much superior, though not so fashionably frequented as others.

The sons of pleasure fly to more genial climes, and court the breezes of the south: and, except those who are allured by connections, and swayed by local considerations, Scarborough contains, among its visitors, more votaries of health than of dissipation.

SITUATION AND GOVERNMENT.

This ancient and populous town lies in the south-east corner of the North Riding of Yorkshire, at the bottom of a beautiful bay, from which it rises in the form of a crescent on the slope of a bold and varied shore, presenting several points of great elevation. It is sheltered from the north-east, by a high and precipitous rock, surrounded by the sea, except on the west. This rock contains on its top a level area of nineteen acres, on which spot stand the ruins of the castle.

Scarborough is distant from London, by the Lincoln road, about 214 miles, and by the road through York 235; from the latter city forty miles. It is a well built and spacious place; but, from its romantic situation, regularity cannot be expected. As in other places of public resort, however, improvements are constantly carrying on here with activity and spirit; and it is now capable of accommodating a large number of visitants of every rank and condition. The range of buildings on the cliff commands a fine view of the castle, town, and a moving scene of ships, with a vast expanse of ocean. The resident inhabitants

Page 354.

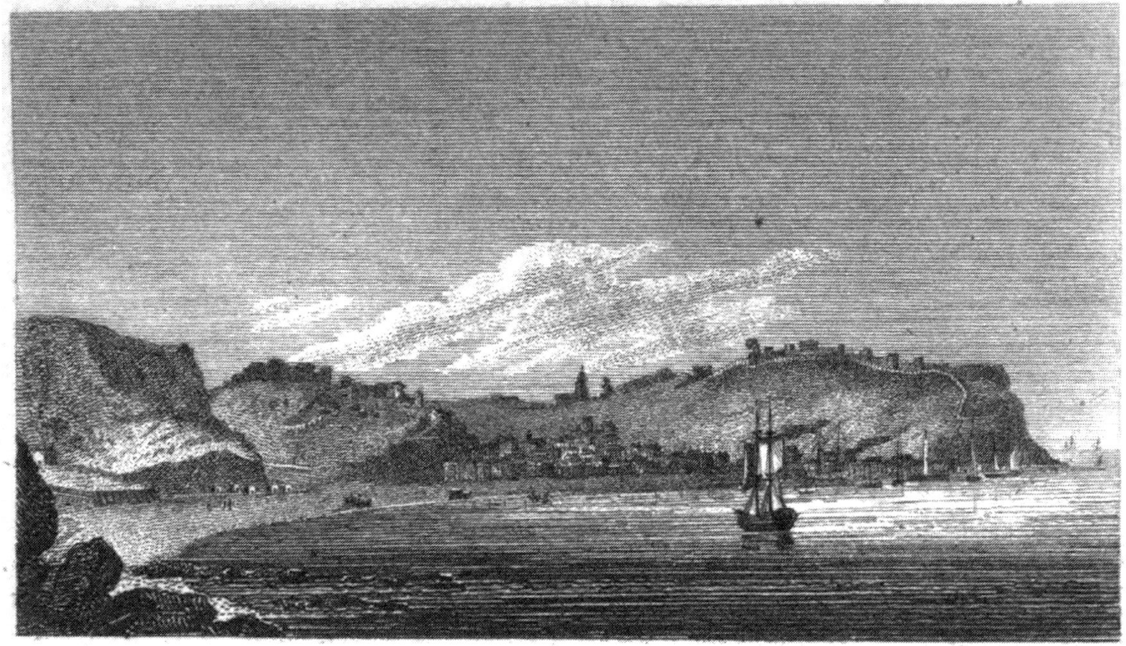

Scarborough.

amount to 7350, many of whom are engaged in maritime concerns.

Scaerburgh, or the town, on the *scar* or cliff, was known to the Saxons. It is a borough and town corporate, governed by two bailiffs, a recorder, two coroners, four chamberlains, and thirty-six common council-men, and returns two members to serve in parliament, which it first began to do in the reign of Edward I.

The first charter of incorporation extant is by Henry II. in the year 1181, but the civic constitution of this place has frequently been changed. The old form of government seems to have been by bailiffs when Richard III. altered it to that of a mayor; but, his charter not being confirmed in council, the bailiffs were restored, and continued till the reign of Charles II. when a mayor was again appointed. In four years, however, the mayor was a second time given up; and, on the accession of William III. the original custom of bailiffs was adopted, and has since been observed without interruption.

THE CASTLE.

Scarborough, as a town, is little known in history, except so far as it is connected with its castle, first founded by William le Gros, Earl of Yorkshire, in the reign of Stephen. On its resumption by the crown, Henry II. very much enlarged and strengthened it; and, from this period it was considered as the key of this important county, and none but persons of high rank and approved fidelity were entrusted with its command.

Edward II. in 1312, when flying before his rebellious nobility, left his minion Piers Gaveston here, as in a place of the greatest security; but, the castle being besieged by Aymer de Valence, Earl of Pembroke, the insolent favorite soon fell a victim to the resentment of the Earl of Warwick.

About 1378, it received great injury from a combined fleet of Scots, French, and Spaniards, under the conduct of one Mercer, who entered the harbour, and carried off several ships. The insult, however, was instantly revenged by Philpot, Alderman of London; who, fitting out a fleet at his own charge, gallantly engaged the enemy, and took their whole armament.

Richard III. added to the original and natural fortifications of this place; but in 1557, Thomas, second son of Lord Stafford, with only thirty-two attendants, arriving from France, surprized and took the castle, which has given rise to the Proverb of "a Scarborough warning." This young nobleman having published a manifesto against the Queen, assumed the title of Lord Protector of England; but, the Earl of Westmoreland collecting some forces, in two days put an end to his dignity.

In the beginning of the civil wars it was garrisoned by the parliament, and the governor having revolted to the king, made a resolute defence for upwards of a year, but at last surrendered on honourable terms, 25th July, 1645. It sustained a second siege of five months in 1648, in favour of the king.

This castle had a stately tower, which serves as a land-mark to mariners, but it was much injured in the conflict between Charles I. and the parliament; the whole now presents a bold picturesque mass of ruins.

In the centre of the line wall, a barrack was erected here about sixty years ago, capable of holding 120 men. There is also an excellent battery of eighteen-pounders.

The air of this spot is remarkably pure and piercing, and from the ruins is a beautiful bird's-eye view of the town, shipping, and the German ocean, which is constantly traversed by innumerable sails.

TRADE.

The pier is very commodious, and the harbour is one of the best in this part of the kingdom, which renders it much resorted to in stormy weather by vessels navigating so dangerous a coast. The ships belonging to the place, are chiefly employed in the Baltic and coal trade. Corn, dried fish, and other articles, are exported coastways. The fisheries for ling, cod, soles, haddocks, turbot, and herrings, are very considerable, and employ many hands. The town and port have about 1500 sea-faring people, who are variously engaged, and, by their different occupations, enliven the scene.

A manufactory of sail-cloth is established in the town, three rope-walks, and several ship-yards, from which are launched vessels as large as 600 tons burthen; so that on the whole, though Scarborough does not depend wholly on its commerce, it cannot be said that it derives all its consequence from the influx of company who resort to its springs and its beach.

BATHING.

The sudden tides and short breakings of the sea, which often come with great impetuosity, and sometimes danger, render it adviseable to employ guides and machines. The machines are about forty, which may give some idea of the numbers that require them. They are well attended, and drawn into any depth the bathers chuse. A boy generally drives the horse, and men and women guides attend if required, in the machines.

The regular charge is a shilling every time, but the attendants expect a gratuity at going away, nearly equal to the sum paid to their masters; and few will dispute their right to a remuneration, when it is considered that they undertake the office from the hopes of receiving one.

Morning, as at other places, is the usual time for bathing, as well as for drinking the waters.

The shore is a fine hard sand; and, during low water, is much frequented by the company for walking or riding.

WARM BATHS.

A very neat and commodious suite of rooms for warm sea-water bathing has been lately established on the cliff by Messrs. Wilson and Travis, surgeons. The terms are 3*s.* for the bath, and 6*d.* for the attendant. Here is likewise a shower-bath, with every necessary accommodation.

THE SPA.

The Spa is about a quarter of a mile south of the town, on the sands, at the foot of a high cliff, and rises upright out of the earth, near the level of the spring-tides, which often overflow it. The Spa consists of two wells, and was discovered about two centuries ago; and ever since, the waters have been held in high estimation.

One of the wells is more purgative, and the other more chalybeate; hence the latter, which is nearest the town, has been called the chalybeate spring, and the other the purgative, though they are both impregnated with different proportions of the same principles. The *aperient* is that which is usually called the Scarborough water. It contains in a gallon, fifty-two grains of calcareous earth, two of ochre, and 266 of vitriolated magnesia. The *chalybeate*, in the same quantity of water, has seventy grains of calcareous earth, 139 of vitriolated magnesia, and eleven of marine salt.

When these waters are poured from one glass into another, they throw up a number of air bubbles, a proof that they contain much fixed air. At the fountain they have both a brisk, pungent, chalybeate taste, but the purgative is also somewhat bitter. From two to four half pints is the quantity usually drank.

These waters are found serviceable in hectic fevers, in weaknesses of the stomach, and indigestion, in all relaxations of the system, nervous, hysteric, and hypochondriacal disorders; in the green-sickness, scurvy, rheumatism, and asthma; in gleets, fluor albus, and other preternatural evacuations; and in habitual costiveness. The manner of varying them, and the best mode of using them, however, must be left to the medical guide.

A person, under the name of governor, resides, during the season, at the Spa, and receives a subscription of 7*s.* 6*d.* each person; one third of which is appropriated to the water-servers, the rest to the corporation. The heat of these springs is between forty-five and forty-six degrees, which is five less than the mean heat of springs in general. From the purgative well, salts are prepared, which are in considerable estimation as a gentle aperient.*

---

* The singular incident that happened in December 1737, whereby this famous Spa had like to have been lost, deserves to be mentioned. The Spa, as before observed, lies about a quarter of a mile from the town, on the sands, and fronting the sea to the east, under a high cliff, the top of which is above the high-water level fifty-four yards. The staith or wharf projecting before the Spa-house, was a large body of stone, bound by timbers, and was a fence against the sea, for the security of the house. It was seventy-six feet long, and fourteen feet high, and in weight, by computation, 2463 tons. The house and buildings were upon a level with the staith, at the north end of which, and near adjoining to it, upon a small rise above the level sands, and at the foot of the stairs that lead up to the top of the said staith, and to the house, were the Spa wells. On Wednesday, December 28, in the morning, a great crack was heard from the cellar of the Spa-house; and, upon search, the cellar was found rent, but, at the time, no farther notice was taken of it. The night following, another crack was heard, and on next Thursday, between two and three in the afternoon, a third, when the top of the cliff behind it rent two hundred and twenty-four yards in length, and thirty-six in breadth, and was all in motion, slowly descending, and so continued till dark. The ground, thus rent, contained about an acre of pasture-land, and had cattle then feeding upon it, but had sunk near seventeen yards perpendicular. The sides of the cliff, nearest the Spa, stood as before, but were rent and broken in many places, and forced forward to the sea about twenty yards. The ground, when sunk, lay upon a level, and the next morning, cattle were still feeding on it, the main land being as a wall on the west, and some part of the side of the cliff as a wall on the east; but the whole to view, gave such a confused prospect, as could hardly be described. The rent of the top of the cliff aforesaid, from the main land, was two hundred and twenty-four yards. The rent con-

LODGINGS, BOARDING-HOUSES, INNS, &c.

Though lodgings are numerous, they are frequently well filled. There is a kind of customary rate of 10*s*. 6*d*. for a room, and half that price for servants apartments; but, as at Bath, the proprietors will not break their suites, while there is any prospect of letting them entire. The principal places where the lodging-houses are situate, are as follow:

On the cliff, most of which have full sea-views, in Harding's-walk, Newborough-street, Long-room-street, Tanner-street, and Queen-street.

There are also two or three Boarding-houses, where persons may board and lodge on reasonable terms. Servants at half price. Provisions of all kinds, particularly fish, are plentiful and cheap at Scarborough. The principal inns are the Black Bull, without the gates; the New Inn, George, and Blue Bell, Newborough; the Blacksmiths' Arms and Talbot, Queen-street; and the Old Globe, St. Sepulchre-

---

tinued from each end, down the side of the cliff, to the sands; was measured on the sands, from one end to the other, one hundred and sixty-eight yards. As the ground sunk, the earth or sand, on which the people used to walk under the cliff, rose upwards out of its natural position, for above one hundred yards in length, on each side of the staith, north and south; and was in some places six, and in others seven yards above its former level. The Spa wells rose with it; but, as soon as it began to rise, the water at the Spa well ceased running, and was gone.

The most rational account then given for this phænomenon is as follows:—The solid earth, sinking on the top of the cliff, as afore-mentioned (which was of so vast a weight, as by computation to amount to 261,360 tons,) pressing gradually upon and into the swampy boggy earth beneath it, would, of course, and did raise the earth and sands, as before noticed, and so effect the mischief we have particularised; but, very luckily for the town, after a diligent search, and clearing away the ruins, they found again the Spa spring, and on trial had the pleasure to perceive the water rather better, than impaired, by the disaster. And now the whole is in a more flourishing condition than ever.

street. All these are posting-houses. Several other persons let horses for hire.

The Coffee-house stands at the corner of Tanner-street, and here the papers may be read for a very moderate subscription.

AMUSEMENTS.

PUBLIC ROOMS.

The Assembly-room is neither distinguished for its beauty nor its elegance, but it is commodious, and sufficient for the reception of a large company. The subscription, for the season, is 1*l.* 1*s.* The rooms are open for dancing on Mondays, Wednesdays, and Fridays. Non-subscribers pay 5*s.* each. Mr. Dormer, the proprietor of the rooms, has opened a subscription-room for newspapers, dinners, &c. on the plan of the London Coffee-houses.

Every gentleman who dances, pays 2*s.* for music; ladies or gentlemen who drink tea, 1*s.*

THEATRE.

The Theatre at this place is neat, and the performers generally masters of their business. To the credit of the company and inhabitants, a taste for the elegant amusements of the stage is very prevalent here.

LIBRARIES.

If ignorance is one of the most dangerous diseases, and "Libraries the treasure of remedies for the soul," Scarborough possesses this antidote in equal perfection with some of its most fashionable rivals.

There are two Circulating Libraries here, the subscription to each of which, for three months, is only 5*s.* and surely it is impossible to lay out that moderate sum more pleasantly or profitably than at one or both of them.

FISHING.

Though numbers in Scarborough make fishing their vocation, the visitors frequently consider it, as well as sailing, among their amusements. The apparatus for fishing in the sea may be readily procured, with proper attendants; and, for those who prefer angling, the Derwent, a mile from the town, presents a favourable opportunity. It abounds in trout, pike, &c. and permission to angle is seldom refused, on application to the proprietors.

GARDENS.

An industrious gardener of this place has laid out his grounds, which are of considerable extent, in walks, which any person, on subscribing *2s. 6d.* may use for the season. The admirers of Flora will find this an inviting lounge, and those who are fond of fruit, may purchase it fresh on the spot.

THE CHURCH.

There is but one church in this large place, and as it rose out of the ruins of one more ancient, which was destroyed in the civil wars, it contains nothing remarkable. In summer, prayers are read every morning. Proper attention is paid to the accommodation of strangers who attend.

Scarborough abounds in Dissenters; Quakers, Presbyterians, Baptists, Methodists, and Roman Catholics, have all their separate places of meeting.

SEAMAN'S HOSPITAL.

This, which is intended for the relief of aged and disabled seamen, is an appendage to, and under the government of, the Trinity-house, London. It is situated on a fine airy hill, in the road towards Peasholme, and affords a comfortable asylum for the objects of its institution. Its funds arise from a rate on ships belonging to the port, and a deduction of *6d.* per month from the pay of their crews.

RIDES AND WALKS ROUND SCARBOROUGH.

The remarkable objects, in the immediate vicinity of Scarborough, are few; yet time never seems to hang heavily on the hands of its visitants. Riding, walking, reading, and music, the Spa,* and the bathing machine, fill up the space which is not devoted to the table or to sleep. The most fashionable promenades are on the sands, both to the north and south of the town. Excursions are frequently made to the following places:

HACKNESS,

The seat of Sir Richard Bempte Johnson, bart. stands in a retired valley, about six miles from Scarborough, and company, who visit the place, are allowed every indulgence they can desire, by the worthy owner.

WYKEHAM.

A spacious house is built here on the site of an old abbey. It belongs to Mr. Langley.

BROMPTON,

The residence of Sir George Cayley, bart. is venerable for having been the residence of that family for many generations.

SCAMPSTON.

This was the favourite residence of the late Sir William St. Quintin. All these places may be seen in a morning's ride; but separately, they possess little that can delay the stranger.

CASTLE HOWARD.

Parties are frequently formed to visit Castle Howard, the seat of the Earl of Carlisle.

* This consists of two wells, hemmed in by a bank, at a considerable expence. They brace and invigorate the stomach, are pleasant to the taste, create an appetite, and are peculiarly serviceable in nervous complaints.

Castle Howard lies twenty-six miles from Scarborough, and is a noble pile of architecture, built under the direction of Sir John Vanburgh. The front is more extensive than Blenheim, which was built by the same architect. The paintings, statues, and other accompaniments, both external and internal, are deservedly admired.

DUNCOMBE PARK.

Though this fine seat, another work of Vanburgh's, lies thirty miles from Scarborough, the visitor seldom regrets his trouble, and the length of his ride. The Duncombe family have long resided here, and they have embellished it with the richest productions of art.

It is impossible, in this place, to describe the beauties of York; but the venerable minster, one of the finest pieces of antient ecclesiastical architecture in the kingdom, will afford a rich gratification to every visitor of taste.

Pl. 32. P. 296

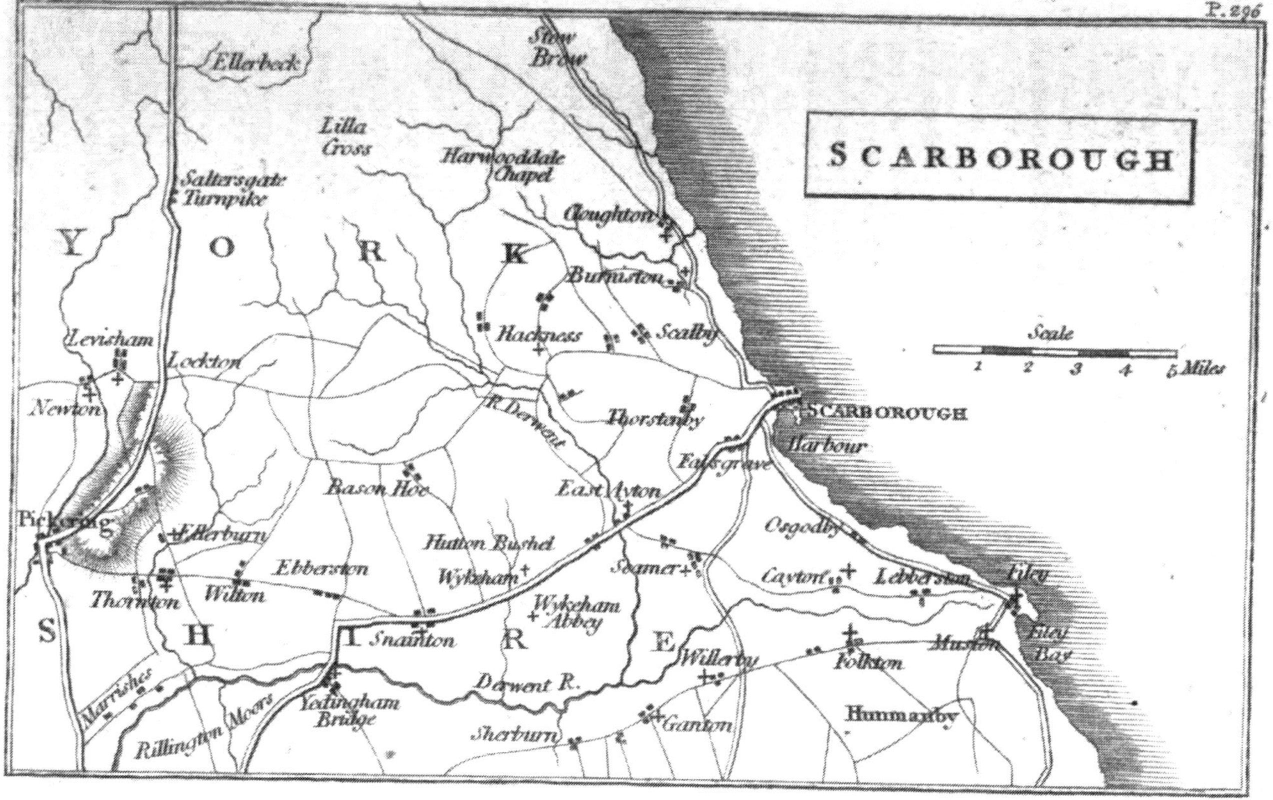
SCARBOROUGH
Scale
1 2 3 4 5 Miles
Y O R K S H I R E
Ellerbeck
Stow Brow
Lilla Cross
Harwooddale Chapel
Saltersgate Turnpike
Cloughton
Burniston
Hackness
Scalby
Levisham
Lockton
Newton
R. Derwent
Thorstonby
SCARBOROUGH
Harbour
Falsgrave
Bason Hoe
East Ayton
Pickering
Ellerburn
Hutton Bushel
Osgodby
Ebberston
Wykeham
Seamer
Cayton
Lebberston
Filey
Thornton
Wilton
Wykeham Abbey
Snainton
Filey Bay
Muston
Willerby
Folkton
Marrishes
Derwent R.
Yedingham Bridge
Hummanby
Rillington Moors
Sherburn
Ganton

SIDMOUTH.

This fashionable watering-place is situate amidst two hills, at the mouth of the little river Sid; on a bay of the English channel, between Exmouth and Lyme Regis, about eleven miles south-east of Exeter.

Though embosomed in this manner by hills, Sidmouth hath yet a fine and extensive prospect of the sea. It was a good sea-port before its harbour was so choaked up with sand, that no ships of burthen could enter it. Leland, who made a survey of the kingdom, in the reign of Henry VIII. thus mentions it; "Sidmouth is a fisschar toun, with a broke of that name, and a bay six miles west of Seton." And Sir William de la Pole, in his account of Devonshire, in the reign of James the First, gives this account of it, "Sidmouth, where the little river Sid runneth into the sea, is a small market-town, and has been famous for fishing." Risdon, in his manuscript Chorographical Survey of Devonshire, thus extends the description: "Since the surrender to the crown, Sidmouth is one of the chiefest fisher towns of this shire, and serveth much provision into the eastern parts; wherein her principal maintenance consists. But in times past it was a port of some account, now choaked with chisel stones and sand, by the vicissitude of the tides."

At present, however, the inhabitants are very badly supplied with fish. But, though Sidmouth has lost in its supplies from the ocean, it has gained, in common with many other places on the coast, by the fashionable rage for bathing. As a watering-place, it is now much frequented, the company every season generally amounting to three hundred. With respect to accommodation, Sidmouth has to boast of an elegant ball-room; and on the beach a commodious tea-room and shed frequented by ladies as well as gentlemen. Neither should we overlook the livery-stables, nearly opposite the London Inn, a neat circular building, with a fountain in the centre. But Sidmouth is not esteemed merely as the resort of people whose pursuit is pleasure. It is also very commonly recommended to invalids, particularly to those who are affected by consumptions; as many of the faculty think this situation equal to the south of France. The inhabitants are remarkable for their healthy appearance, and for their longevity. Such, indeed, might be naturally expected, from the salubrity of the air, the fine dry soil, and a situation the most delicious, open to the ocean, yet not subject to fogs, and screened from all but the southern winds.

The rides and walks about Sidmouth are very pleasant, and at every turn present a variety of romantic and beautiful views. The scenery on the coast to Seaton is remarkably pleasing and picturesque, and is esteemed the finest on the western shores of Devon. At Otterton, about three miles distant, is the seat of Lord Rolle.

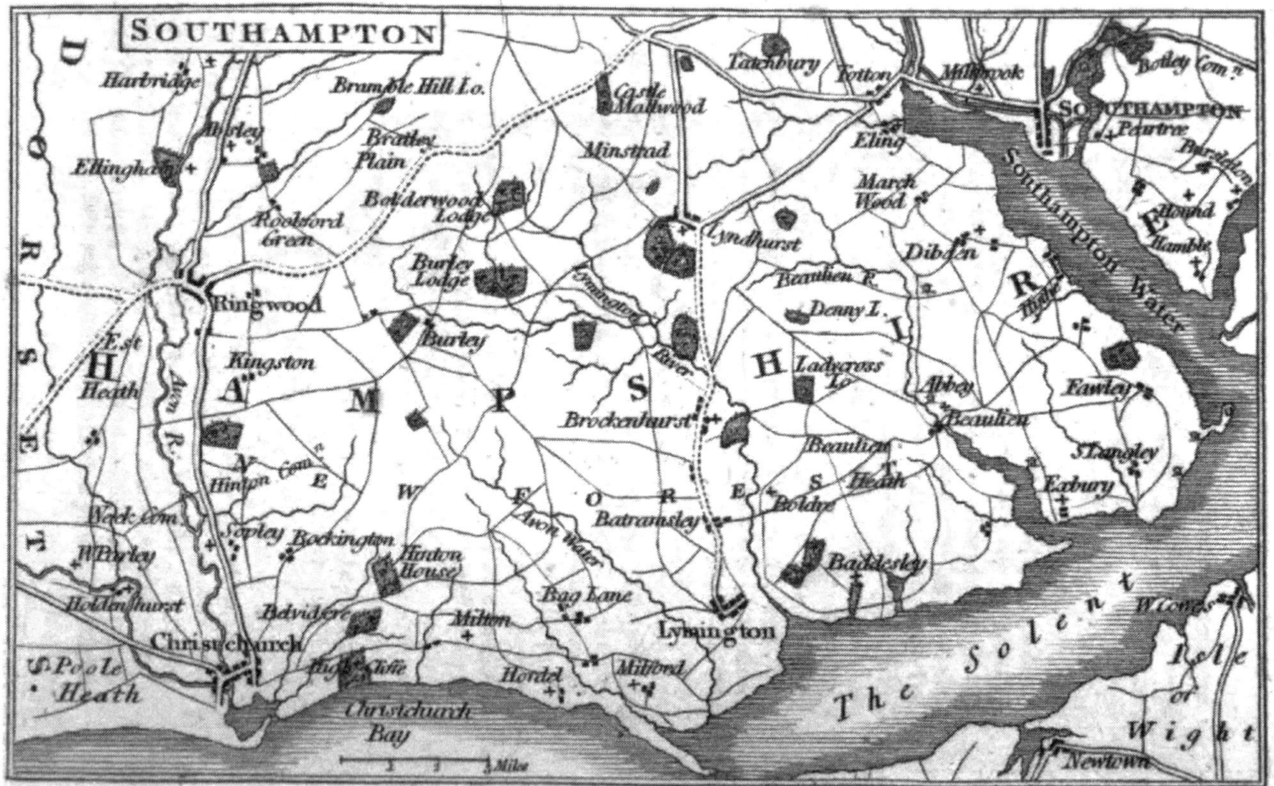
SOUTHAMPTON
Harbridge
Bramble Hill Lo.
Castle Malwood
Tatchbury
Totton
Southampton
Ellingham
Bratley Plain
Minstead
Eling
Bolderwood Lodge
March Wood
Rockford Green
Lyndhurst
Dibden
Burley Lodge
Beaulieu R.
Denny L.
Southampton Water
Hamble
Ringwood
Burley
Kingston
Ladycross Lo.
Abbey
Fawley
Brockenhurst
Beaulieu
Batramsley
Avon Water
Baddesley
Hinton House
Bag Lane
Belvidere
Milton
Lymington
Christchurch
Poole Heath
Hordel
Milford
Christchurch Bay
The Solent
Isle of Wight
Newtown
3 Miles

SOUTHAMPTON.

The lovely situation of Southampton, the elegance of its buildings, the amenity of its environs, and the various other attractions which it possesses, in a very high degree, will always render it a place of fashionable residence, as well as of frequent resort. The beach, on which are several bathing machines, is very favourable for the purpose; and the sea-water here is as salt as that at the Needles. The air is soft and mild, and sufficiently impregnated with saline particles to render it agreeable, and even salutary, to those who cannot endure a full exposure to the sea, on a bleak and open shore.

SITUATION.

Equally adapted for health, pleasure, and commerce. Southampton, distant about seventy-seven miles from London, is bounded on the east by the river Itchin, and on the west by the Tese or Anton, which rises near Whitchurch. It occupies a kind of peninsula, the soil of which is a hard gravel; and, as the buildings rise from the water with a gentle ascent, the streets are always clean and dry. The approach from the London road is uncommonly striking; in fact, it is almost unparallelled in the beauty of its features, for the space of two miles. At first appear an expanse of water, and the distant Isle of Wight, the charming scenery of the New Forest, and Southampton itself, in pleasing perspective. Elegant seats and rows of trees, nearer the town, line the road on both sides; and, on entering the place, by one of its most fashionable streets, that venerable remain of antiquity the Bargate, gives a finish to the scene, and fixes the impression of the objects through which we have passed.

SKETCH OF ITS ANCIENT HISTORY.

So commanding was this situation that the Romans, who always selected with taste and judgment, had a station in this vicinity. The present Bittern, lying about two miles from Southampton, on the Itchin, was undoubtedly the site of the ancient Clausentum, as has been satisfactorily proved by the remains of walls, and the frequent discovery of Roman coins.

When, or on what occasion Clausentum was destroyed, is wholly unknown. The opposite side of the river, offering advantages and conveniences which Clausentum did not possess, might probably be a principal cause of its desertion, and of the rise of Southampton, anciently Hantun, supposed to have been derived from An or Ant, the British name of the river and estuary, and tun or ton, a town. South was doubtless added to distinguish it from North Hamton.

It is not improbable, indeed, that Southampton was a place of some note among the Britons; but the first authentic accounts we now possess of it, commence in the ninth century. During the invasions of the Danes, who infested the English coasts for almost two centuries, this place was more than once ravaged by them: and in 838, under the reign of Ethelwolf, these formidable pirates, with a fleet of thirty-three gallies, landed here, and committed horrible devastations; but, at last, Wolphard, the governor of the country, defeated and drove them to their ships.

In the year 981, they landed again, and committed their usual enormities; and, about twelve years after, headed by Sweyn, King of Denmark, and Olave, King of Norway, they repeated their former cruelties and devastations. Emboldened, however, by the pusillanimity of Ethelred, they did not, on this occasion, confine themselves to the sea-coast, but seizing all the horses they could find, they car-

Page 368

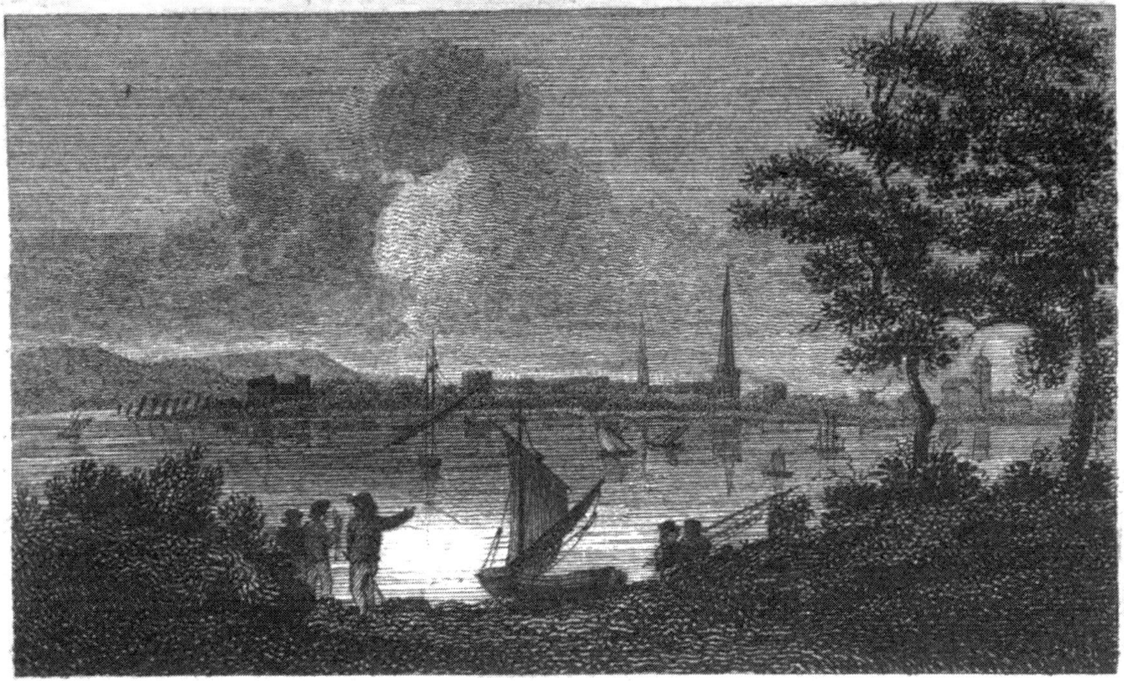

Southampton.

ried the terror of their arms into the inland counties; and, such was the weakness of the English, that they were glad to buy off the two leaders, with a promised reward of 16,000*l.* and, till this sum could be raised, Sweyn and Olave sat down unmolested, at Southampton.

All the exertions of Edmund Ironside were unable to recover what the imbecility of his predecessors had lost; and, after repeated contests, he was compelled to yield up half his kingdom to the Danish leader, Canute.

In this barbarian, for in no other light can the Danes at that period be considered, there were qualities that raised him above the level of chieftains of his age and nation. He was gallant and enterprising, and endowed with a considerable share of good sense and penetration.

It was on the beach of Southampton that he gave a memorable proof of the justness of his sentiments. His courtiers vieing with each other in their adulation, one of them exclaimed, that there was nothing beyond the reach of his power. Canute, disgusted with this hyperbolical compliment, ordered a chair to be carried to the sea-shore, when the tide was coming in; and, having seated himself near the edge of the water, in all the insignia of royalty, surrounded by his attendants, he commanded the waves to retire, and to obey the voice of him whose authority knew no bounds. The tide, observing its natural course, gradually approached, and at last began to wash his feet: when starting up, he reproached his courtiers for their servile flattery, and observed, "that the most powerful-created being was but weak and impotent, when compared with the lord of the universe, with whom alone omnipotence resided, and who could say to the ocean, *thus far shalt thou go, and no farther.*" From this time, it is said, he never wore a crown.

So completely had the ravages of the Danes reduced the inhabitants, and diminished the consequence of Southampton, that in the survey which the conqueror ordered to be taken, we find it contained only seventy-nine men in demesne, though it was then a burgh, a proof of its being a place of some importance in the Anglo-saxon times.

Henry II. gave it the first charter of incorporation, which was confirmed by subsequent monarchs. King John gave the farm of Southampton, with the port of Portsmouth, to the burgesses of the former town, in consideration of an annual payment, into the exchequer, of 200*l.* by weight.

With such powers and privileges, Southampton began to increase in wealth and commerce. A brisk wine trade was carried on with France; the stannaries were removed hither, and the port revenue rose to a considerable sum.

Indeed, the jurisdiction of the port of Southampton was so extensive, by the grants it enjoyed, that the burgesses were liable to constant invasions of their rights, from the neighbouring maritime towns. In the reign of Edward II. an action was brought against Lymington, for having taken duties on salt, barley, and oats to the amount of 40*s*. and customs on cloth to the amount of 100*s*. The mayor and burgesses of Southampton averred, that they held their town, with the port, extending from beyond Hurst to Langstone, of the crown, at 220*l.* per ann. and this claim the jury confirmed, and gave them adequate damages.

After rising in prosperity for some ages, Southampton received a sudden check in the reign of Edward III. during the contest which arose between Philip de Valois and that prince, about the right of succession to the French monarchy. A French fleet, of fifty gallies, sailed up Southampton river in 1338; and, after plundering the inhabitants, reduced a considerable part of the town to ashes. They did not, however, effect this with impunity. The son of the King of Sicily, and several distinguished persons of their party, were slain, and the remainder obliged to take shelter on board their ships.

The inhabitants, on recovering from their consternation, began to rebuild the town, and to supply it with double ditches, strong walls, and watch-towers. Richard II. added a lofty castle, raised on an artificial mount, for the defence of the harbour; and, from this period, Southampton seems to have been protected from foreign violence.

It was here that the gallant army, which gained immortal honour in the field of Agincourt, assembled, before its embarkation, in 1415. The spot on which it encamped, called West-quay, is now covered with water.

While Henry V. was waiting at this place for a favourable wind, a conspiracy was formed, which, had it not been detected, must have ruined all his plans. The Earl of Cambridge, Lord Scrope, and Sir Thomas Grey, were the principal conspirators. It is generally supposed that they were bribed by the French court, to assassinate Henry, and though the authority of Shakespeare will be thought doubtful evidence, yet it must be supposed that he spoke the current belief.

See you my princes, and my noble peers,
These English monsters! My Lord Cambridge here!
You know how apt our love was to accord
To furnish him with all appertinents
Belonging to his honour: and this man
Hath, for a few light crowns, lightly conspir'd,
And sworn unto the practices of France,
To kill us here in Hampton: to the which
This knight, no less for bounty bound to us
Than Cambridge is, hath likewise sworn:
    But oh!
What shall I say to thee, Lord Scrope?
    Thou cruel,
Ingrateful, savage, and inhuman creature!

Hen. V. Act. ii. Scene 2.

The conspirators were speedily tried, condemned, and executed, at this place; and their remains interred in the chapel of God's House, where the following inscription may be seen, on a monument, by a predecessor of the present Lord Delaware.

RICHARD EARL OF CAMBRIDGE,
LORD SCROPE OF MASHAM,
SIR THOMAS GREY OF NORTHUMBERLAND,
CONSPIRED
TO MURDER KING HENRY V. IN THIS TOWN,
AS HE WAS PREPARING TO SAIL WITH HIS ARMY
AGAINST CHARLES VI. KING OF FRANCE;
FOR WHICH CONSPIRACY THEY WERE EXECUTED,
AND BURIED NEAR THIS PLACE.
IN THE YEAR, MCCCCXV.

When the feuds between the houses of York and Lancaster raged, during the reign of Edward IV. a fierce skirmish between the partizans of the Red and White Roses broke out here, in which several of the inhabitants fell. The Yorkists being at length victorious, Edward, hastening to Southampton, caused the prisoners to be impaled; an instance of vengeance that reflects eternal disgrace on that monarch.

When Leland, the antiquary, was making his perambulation of England, to search the conventual libraries, he visited Southampton, of which he gives this account:

"There be in the fair and right strong wall of New Hampton, eight gates. Over Bar-gate by North, is the *Domus civica*, and under it is the town prison. There is a great suburb, and a great double dyke, well watered, on each hand, without it. The East-gate is strong, not so large as Bar-gate, and in its suburb stands St. Mary's church. To the South-gate joins a Castelet,* well ordinanced to be at that quarter of the haven. There is another mean gate, a little farther south, called God's House-gate, of an hospital, founded by two merchants, joined to it; and not far beyond it is Water-gate, without which is

* This is still standing; but, as the vicinity to Portsmouth, and the strength of our marine, render it no longer necessary, as a defence, it is converted into a prison for debtors. Near it, on a plat-form, is a single piece of ordinance, but a very beautiful one, given to the town by Henry VIII.

a quay; West-gate is strong, and has a quay without it. There are two more gates. The glory of the castle is in the dungeon, which is both large, fair, and strong, both by work and the site of it.

"There be five parish churches in the town. Holy-rood church standeth in the chief street, which is one of the fairest streets that is in any town in England, and is well built, for timber building. There be many fair merchants houses, and in the south-east part was a college of Grey Friars. Here was also an hospital, called God's-house, founded by two merchants, impropriated since to Queen's College, Oxford."

PRESENT STATE.

Southampton now exhibits a very different appearance from what it did in the time of Leland.—The High-street, however, still continues to maintain the pre-eminence which he assigned it, but the "timber buildings" have disappeared, and brick has chiefly been substituted. In its width, bend, and beauty, it greatly resembles the High-street of Oxford; but is superior to it in its commencement with the Bar, and its termination with the quay.

Near Holy-rood church, in going down the street, a beautiful view of the river, and New Forest, opens by the removal of the Water-gate, and the adjacent houses on the east; and this view improves as you approach the quay.

In this street are shops, which may vie with any in London, and here apartments are frequently let to summer visitants, which are equally pleasant and commodious. Conduits, disposed at proper distances, supply it with excellent water, which is brought from a considerable distance, by pipes; and, except in the eastern part of the town towards St. Mary's, the streets are well paved and lighted, and regularly patroled by watchmen.

Many new and elegant piles of building have arisen within the last few years. Albion-place, Moira-place, Brunswick-place, and various other assemblages, do honour to the taste and opulence of their projectors and proprietors. The population has increased in a similar degree, and amounts to nearly 10,000 souls.

TRADE AND IMPROVEMENTS.

The principal trade of Southampton is with Portugal, for wine and fruit, and with the islands of Jersey, Guernsey, Alderney, and Sark. Several sloops are continually passing and repassing between those islands and Southampton, which, exclusive of goods, carry away annually a limited quantity of unwrought wool, which, by act of parliament, must be sent from, or relanded and duty paid at this port. In return they import large quantities of coarse worsted hose.

There is, likewise, during peace, a frequent communication between Southampton and Havre de Grace. The merchants have also some vessels engaged in the Baltic trade; and the corn, wine, and timber-merchants of Southampton are both numerous and respectable. Silk manufactories are established here; and, at South Stoneham, a few miles distant, are mills for manufacturing blocks and pumps for the navy, the invention of Mr. Walter Taylor, who has an exclusive patent for their fabrication.

To facilitate the communication between Southampton and Salisbury, an act of parliament was obtained in 1795, for cutting a canal from the platform at Southampton, to join the Andover navigation at Red-bridge; and, likewise, a cut from Northam to Houndwell, adjoining Southampton, to connect with the Winchester navigation.

The present Poet Laureat's Epigram, on this subject, is ingenious, and will not soon be forgotten.

Southampton's wise sons found their river so large,
Though 'twould carry a ship, 'twould not carry a barge;

So wisely determin'd to cut by its side
A stinking canal, where small vessels might glide.
Like the man, who contriving a hole in his wall,
To admit his two cats—the one large t'other small,—
When a great hole was cut for the first to go through,
Would a little one have, for the little cat too.

In his Naucratia, too, the same author has vented his indignation with the enthusiasm of genius:

O Milbrook* ! shall my devious feet no more
Pace the smooth margin of thy pebbly shore !—
Now through the stagnant pool, by banks confin'd,
Rolls the slow barge, dragg'd by th' inglorious hind,—
By vengeance arm'd, ye powers of ocean rise !
And when full orb'd in equinoctial skies
The pale moon hangs, and, with malignant pride,
Rouses the driving storm, and swells the tide,
Lift high the trident, and with giant blow,
Lay of vain man the pigmy labours low;
Chastise the weak presumption that would chain
The briny surge, and subjugate the main!

But though much may be allowed to poets, there are not wanting strong arguments in favour of the canal to Redbridge, the river at times not being navigable, on account of the wind, for days together.

We mention, however, with pleasure and applause, a real improvement of another kind. A bridge has been thrown over the Itchin at Northam, and another over the Bursledon river, by which the road to Portsmouth has been shortened several miles, and the necessity of ferrying across, in a great measure, obviated.

CORPORATION, MARKETS, &C.

All former charters granted to Southampton were confirmed by Charles I. The corporation consists of a mayor, a recorder, a sheriff, and two bailiffs; those only who have served one of those offices are common-council-men. The burgesses, however, are unlimited, and in consequence of their election have

* Where H. J. Pye, esq. formerly resided.

a vote for a mayor and members of parliament.—Among the burgesses are commonly some of the royal family. At present his Majesty, the Prince of Wales, the Dukes of York, Cumberland, Cambridge, and Gloucester, honour the list. All who have passed the chair are aldermen, and there are eleven justices of the peace, namely, the mayor for the time being, the Bishop of Winchester, the recorder, the last mayor, the five aldermen, and two burgesses. Other officers are, the town-clerk, four serjeants at mace, a town crier, &c.

In the mayor's bailiff's court small debts are recovered. In the Guildhall, where the quarter-sessions are held, all causes are tried; not excepting capital crimes, for which, however, a special commission must be taken out.

Henry VI. made Southampton a county in itself. The mayor is admiral of the liberties from Langstone Harbour to Hurst-castle, and half-seas over from Calshot-castle to the Isle of Wight. There are nearly 600 voters for members of parliament for this place.

Four annual fairs are held here. Trinity fair commences on Saturday in Whitsun week, and continues till Wednesday following, with several singular ceremonies and observances. St. Mark's fair is held on the 6th and 7th of May. The others, which are inconsiderable, are on Tuesday after old St. Andrew's day, and Tuesday before Shrove Tuesday.

There are three weekly market-days, Tuesday, Thursday, and Saturday, when meat, fish, butter, vegetables, and other kinds of provisions, are plentiful; various species of fish, such as cod, sole, salmon, smelts, mullet, plaice, flounders, may be purchased here frequently on reasonable terms.

The market-house is a large modern fabric: and over it is the council-chamber of the corporation, a very elegant apartment.

RELIGIOUS EDIFICES, &c.

Formerly a college of Grey Friars stood in the south-east part of the town. The hospital, called God's House, is a very ancient foundation, built, as it is said, by Gervasius and Protisius, two brothers, and merchants. In process of time it was impropriated to Queen's College, Oxford, on condition that a certain number of poor scholars, of that college, should be maintained from a fund of surplusages.

The society at present consists of a warden, four old men, and as many women, who, besides their lodging, are allowed two shillings a week each, and under the will of Mrs. Fifield, they have an annual allowance of coals.

The adjoining French Chapel was appropriated, about the year 1567, for the Walloon Protestants. Its congregation, however, now consists chiefly of persons from the islands of Jersey and Guernsey. Service is performed according to the rites of the Church of England, but in the French language.

There are six parishes, though but five churches, at Southampton, viz. Holy-rood, St. Michael, All Saints, St. Lawrence and St. John, and St. Mary.

HOLY-ROOD CHURCH.

This is a vicarage belonging to Queen's College, Oxford, worth about 200*l.* per annum. It has a fine organ, and several handsome monuments, particularly one by Rysbrack, to the memory of Miss E. Stanley, with the following inscription, by the author of the Seasons.

Here Stanley, rest! escap'd this mortal strife,
Above the joys, beyond the woes of life.
Fierce pangs no more thy lively beauties stain,
And sternly try thee with a year of pain.
No more, sweet Patience, feigning oft relief,
Light thy sick eye to cheat a parent's grief:

With tender heart to save her anxious groan,
No more thy bosom presses down its own.
Now well-earn'd peace is thine, and bliss sincere,
Ours be the lenient, not unpleasing tear.

O born to bloom, then sink beneath the storm!
To shew us virtue in her fairest form;
To shew us artless Reason's mortal reign,
What boastful science arrogates in vain:
Th' obedient passions, knowing each the part,
Calm light the head, and harmony the heart.

Yes, we must follow soon, will glad obey,
When a few suns have roll'd their cares away:
Tir'd with vain life, will close the willing eye;
'Tis the great birthright of mankind to die!
Blest be the breeze that wafts us to the shore,
Where death-divided friends shall part no more,
To join thee there, here with thy dust repose,
Is all the hope thy hapless mother knows.

Born 1720. Died 1738.

J. THOMSON.

ST. MICHAEL'S.

This church has a high, slender, octagonal spire, which serves as a mark for ships entering the harbour. Here the new mayor is always sworn into his office. Here is a monument, erected, as is supposed, to a female of the Wriothesley family, but the inscription round the canopy is nearly obliterated.

ALL SAINTS,

Is an elegant modern structure, which does honour to its architect, Mr. Reveley, cramped as his energies are said to have been, in the prosecution of the plan.

It fronts the High-street, and is adorned with four three-quarter columns of the Ionic order, each thirty-six feet high, crowned with an ample pediment. The angles of the front, which is sixty-six feet wide, are finished on each side with Grecian pilasters. Around the church runs an entablature, supported on each flank with similar pilasters, standing on a plain basement, without any projection. The south side is lighted by sixteen windows, in two ranges: the north, abutting on houses, has no windows.

The interior dimensions are ninety-five feet in length, and sixty-one in breadth; the height from the pavement to the cieling, forty-seven feet. A spacious gallery surrounds three sides of the church. Neither columns nor protruding beams are used to support this ample roof. Arched catacombs occupy the substruction of the building, where the right of burial is purchased of the parish.

The turret at the east end is wholly unworthy of the noble edifice to which it belongs. It is scarcely large enough to support the clock on a nobleman's stable. But this defect, we have been assured, does not rest with Reveley.

ST. LAWRENCE.

This is a small church in the High-street, and has nothing remarkable. The parish of St. John was united to this in 1706, and the church of the latter was pulled down.

ST. MARY'S.

This valuable benefice, which is a precentorship, is in the gift of the Bishop of Winchester, and is worth 1400*l.* per annum. The present rector is the Rev. Francis North, son of the Bishop. The church-yard is the principal burying-ground here, and contains numerous tombs and inscriptions.

SCHOOLS.

A grammar-school was founded here by Edward VI. and is in high repute. Here are, likewise, private schools for young ladies and gentlemen, which are said to be excellently conducted; and no situation can be finer than Southampton, for the health and education of youth.

CHARITIES.

Thorner's alms-houses for poor widows, at the entrance of the town, are an elegant structure, erected in 1789.

Alderman Taunton's charity-school for educating and apprenticing poor boys, is also an excellent foundation. Out of the produce of the estate bequeathed by him, 40*l.* is yearly appropriated to the apportioning female servants on their marriage, who have lived four years at least in a reputable family, and with a fair character. There are other charities, but of no particular consequence to be noticed here.

BAR-GATE,

The principal, and formerly the only approach by land, is a splendid remnant of the fortifications of this place. The north front, which is supposed to have been erected in the reign of Edward III. is semi-octagonal, flanked with two lower semi-circular turrets, and crowned with large and handsome open machicolations. The arch of entrance, which is long and deep, is highly pointed, and adorned with mouldings. Above the arch, on a row of sunk pannels, alternately square and oblong, is a shield in relief, charged with the arms of England, Scotland, Paulet, Tylney, Abdy, Noel, Mill, Wyndham, &c. These arms, however, are not of ancient date, and from a minute inspection of the component parts of this curious gate, Sir Henry Englefield is of opinion that the internal centre could not have been erected later than the early Norman times.

The front towards the High-street is modern, plain, and uninteresting, except that in a central niche it contains a whole-length statue of Queen Anne.

Over the arches of the two foot and carriage-ways, is a Town-hall, fifty-two feet by twenty-one, with which a room for the grand jury communicates. The windows in these apartments bear marks of antiquity.

From the leads, the whole of this noble gate may be traced, and a great part of the town may be seen. Two lions sejent, cast in lead, guard the entrance of Bargate, and on this side are likewise two gigantic figures, representing Ascupart and Sir Bevois of Southampton, his redoubted conqueror, according to the following couplet:

Bevois conquer'd Ascupart, and after slew the boare,
And then he cross'd beyond the seas to combat with the More.

WALLS.

In some places the ancient walls are quite destroyed, and only an antiquary can trace their course; in others they still present a venerable appearance. Fronting the area of the public baths and rooms, they are of a great height, and exhibit a peculiar mode of building, and, though very ornamental, little calculated for defence or security. Towers appear to have been erected at certain distances, several of which still remain. The whole circuit of the walls is computed to be a mile and a quarter, though the present town cannot be less than three miles round.

THE CASTLE, &c.

This stands near the middle of the south part of the town. From the High-street, the approach to it is up Castle-lane. The area of the castle seems to have been of a semicircular form, of which the town wall to the sea, formed the diameter. The keep stood on a high artificial mount, and from its ruins a small round tower has been constructed, from the leads of which there is a delightful bird's-eye view of Southampton, and of the environs, lying like a map before the eye of the spectator.

"The high mount, and circular form of the

keep," says Sir H. Englefield, "indicate an antiquity much higher than the time of Richard II. who probably only repaired and strengthened the castle." This ingenious antiquary seems to think it of Saxon origin. The Marquis of Lansdowne lately made a purchase of the castle, for the purpose of converting into a residence for himself; and the additions to the original building are now very considerable and extensive. His lordship also bought many houses near to the castle, several of which were taken down to enable him to complete his plan of improvements.

In Porter's-lane, at the bottom of the High-street, Sir H. Englefield discovered a building which he conjectures was originally a palace. It is evidently of great antiquity, and was probably inhabited by the Saxon or Danish kings, who occasionally made Southampton their residence.

LODGINGS, BOARDING-HOUSES, INNS, &c.

In every part of Southampton, lodgings may be hired, from a whole house to a single apartment. During the season, which commences in July and ends in October, the terms are often high; but, since other sea-bathing places have started up in every direction on our coasts, as the influx of company must be less at each, the expences are more nearly equalized.

The accommodations at the boarding-houses are good, and the society pleasant and select. Harland's hotel is an excellent house.

The Star, Coach and Horses, George, Dolphin, Vine and Mitre, are all capital houses of entertainment. At the George, a coffee-room is fitted up, well furnished with newspapers. The terms of admission are: Yearly subscribers, 1*l.* 1*s.* quarterly 6*s.* monthly 2*s.* 6*d.* non-subscribers 3*d.* each time.

BATHS.

Near the west quay is a range of convenient and

permanent baths for ladies and gentlemen, rented by Mr. Chilton. The water is changed every tide; and, though it contains less salt than where the tide is pure and unmixed, it does not appear to be less efficacious in those complaints for which cold sea-bathing is generally prescribed.

Here is also a commodious warm bath, which may be engaged for any hour. Terms 3*s.* 6*d.* each time.

Further on towards the channel are Mr. Goodman's baths, commodious and well frequented, and particularly adapted for those who wish to learn to swim.

Each suite of baths is provided with every necessary convenience, and the whole is laid out in a judicious and elegant manner. Careful guides attend each bath.

In addition to these accommodations for bathing, Mr. Cole has lately constructed bathing-machines, at the Cross-house, near Itchin-ferry, which meet with encouragement.

CHALYBEATE SPRING.

At the bottom of Orchard-street, on the right, without Bargate, is a spring, of the nature of Tunbridge-wells, and is used with effect in the same complaints for which that chalybeate is recommended. A middle-sized tumbler is a sufficient dose, which it is more adviseable to repeat than enlarge. This water is frequently drank to promote the advantages of a course of sea-bathing.

PUBLIC ROOMS.

The public rooms are situate near the baths, and command a delightful prospect of Southampton river, and the sylvan scenery of the opposite shore.

The ball-room is spacious, and handsomely decorated. The band of music is disposed in the centre. The card-rooms, and other appendages, are corresponding to the stile of the rest.

Mr. Martin, the proprietor of these rooms, fitted them up at a liberal expence; and no convenience seems wanting, except an easier approach for carriages, for which the situation is unfavourable.

A minute attention to dress is not required here; but the following regulations, established by W. Lynne, esq. master of the ceremonies, must be complied with:

REGULATIONS.

May 24th, 1797.

At a meeting of the subscribers held this day, the following regulations were established at these rooms:

I. That the rooms be opened every day in the week, Sundays excepted.

II. That there be undress balls on Tuesday and Saturday nights, and that the subscribers to the ball are to pay, gentlemen 1*l.* 1*s.* ladies 10*s.* 6*d.* for the season.

III. That non-subscribers pay 5*s.* admission to each ball.

IV. That on Saturday nights the rooms be opened for card-assemblies and promenades. Dancing to be permitted. Non-subscribers to pay 1*s.* each admittance.

N. B. Children of all ages are subject to the above regulations.

The master of the ceremonies respectfully requests that non-subscribers will afford him an opportunity, on their entrance to the rooms, of being presented to them, that he may be enabled to shew them that attention it is so much his wish to observe.

Extract from the proceedings of the committee, January 28th, 1786. "That the master of the ceremonies shall be supported in the execution of his office, by all the subscribers at large; and, any misbehaviour shewn to him, shall be considered as done to the whole company,"

W. LYNNE, M. C.

PRICE OF CARDS.

	s.	d.
Two packs for whist, quadrille, cribbage, casino, and all games not here specified	10	0
Ditto one pack - - -	6	0
Commerce and vingt et un - -	9	0
Loo - - - - - -	8	6
If more than eight play, each - -	1	0
Lottery - - - - -	10	6
After the first packs, at any game, per pack	4	6

Southampton, May 24, 1797.

It being absolutely necessary in all polite assemblies to establish some regulations, without which no order or decorum can be preserved—the company are respectfully requested to comply with the following:

I. That no precedence take place at these rooms, after the balls are begun.

II. That the balls shall begin precisely at eight o'clock, and finish at twelve.

III. That ladies and gentlemen who dance down a country dance, shall not quit their places till the dance is finished, unless they mean to dance no more that night.

IV. That after a lady has called a dance, and danced it down, her place in the next dance is at the bottom.

The prevailing custom of ladies allowing their acquaintances to stand above them in the set, having been the origin of much dispute, and a material interruption to the dance, the master of the ceremonies would think himself highly blameable to suffer it to continue. It is his intention to be extremely attentive to prevent it in future.

V. That gentlemen are not to appear at the rooms in boots.

VI. That no tea-table be carried into the card-room on ball-nights.

As it is the wish of the master of the ceremonies that all improper company should be kept from these rooms, he respectfully requests that all strangers, as well ladies as gentlemen, to whom he has not the honour to be personally known, will offer him some occasion of being presented to them, to enable him to shew that attention and respect to every individual resorting to this place, which he will be ever studious to observe.

W. LYNNE, M. C.

There is a ball at these rooms, annually on the 4th of June, in honour of his Majesty's birth-day, and the rooms open the beginning of July, at which time the season is said to commence, and the balls are continued on Tuesdays, Thursdays, and Saturdays, till the close of the season, the latter end of October. The master of the ceremonies has two balls during the season, one in the month of August, and the other in October.

THE WINTER ASSEMBLIES.

These assemblies are held at the Dolphin inn, and were at first established in 1785. Assemblies are held every fortnight during the winter, on Tuesdays, commencing the beginning of November, and ending in April; at which, by the unanimous desire of the subscribers, W. Lynne, esq. acts as master of the ceremonies, with a clear ball on any one night during the season, most eligible to himself, the queen's ball-night alone excepted.

Rules and Regulations.

The rules and regulations are nearly the same as at the summer-balls, with this difference;

I. That the balls shall commence at seven o'clock, and finish precisely at eleven.

II. That all surplus of money arising from the subscription be appropriated for the purpose of the assembly only.

III. That each subscriber shall pay 1*s*. 6*d*. admission, and non-subscribers 3*s*.

IV. That all non-subscribers, as well as all new subscribers, previous to their admission, be introduced to the master of the ceremonies, by a subscriber.

V. That each person pay 6*d*. for tea on admission.

RATES OF CHAIRS.

I. From the rooms to any part below the gate, 9*d*. to any part above the gate, 1*s*.

II. From any part within the gates, 9*d*. without the gates, 1*s*.

III. For every chair kept longer than ten minutes, 6*d*. and so on for every half hour afterwards.

IV. Double fare to stop and get out; if only stop a short time and get out, but single fare.

V. From any part above the gate to Moira-place, 1*s*. if below the gate, 1*s*. 6*d*.

VI. From St. Mary's, or Orchard-lane, to any part of the town, 1*s*. 6d.

VII. From above Bar to the Quay, 1*s*. 3*d*.

All these fares are double after eleven o'clock a night.

THEATRE.

A theatre was built here by subscription in 1766, but though afterwards enlarged and improved, it was at last found so inconvenient, that Mr. Collins, the manager, was induced to purchase St. John's Hospital, on the site of which a capacious and elegant theatre has been erected. The company, which is very respectable, open their campaign in August or September, and perform every Monday, Wednesday, and Friday, till the end of October, after which they take a regular circuit to Portsmouth, Chichester, and Winchester, from whence they return to this place.

MISCELLANEOUS AMUSEMENTS.

For the amusement of gentlemen, there are Billiard tables and a fives-court; and also a pleasant bowling-green, near the plat-form, which is well filled in a summer's evening.

The principal promenade is above Bar-street, towards the barracks, which is often filled with beauty and fashion. The walk round the beach, on the margin of what is termed the Southampton water, is much frequented on account of its airiness and picturesque scenery.

For riding and walking, indeed, in every direction, there is the greatest inducement in this vicinity, as the roads are most excellent, and for some miles round, lead to a succession of pleasing or magnificent objects.

No amusement, however, which Southampton affords, can be more salutary or delightful than sailing. A boat, or pleasure-vessel, may be engaged for hours, or by the day, in any course, on reasonable terms; while the packets, which daily sail to Cowes,* and receive passengers at 1*s.* each, offer a cheap and agreeable aquatic excursion, which is frequently enjoyed by the company resorting to this place. Packets and hoys likewise sail from Southampton to Portsmouth, to Guernsey and Jersey, and in time of peace to Havre de Grace, in France.

LIBRARIES.

Baker and Fletcher's Library, in the High-street, contains a well-chosen collection of more than 7000 volumes, in every branch of learning, and every department of composition. Jewellery, stationary, &c. are likewise sold at this shop.

These gentlemen have also a printing-office, from which books have issued that would do no discredit to the London press. The good sense, information, and civility, of this family, render their acquaintance desirable to every visitor of the place.

* For the picturesque features of this voyage, see COWES.

Skelton's library, standing nearly opposite, is likewise well filled with valuable and entertaining books, and is much frequented.

He has likewise a printing-office, and a subscription news-room, which is open from nine in the morning to nine in the evening, on reasonable terms.

There are some other libraries in Southampton, which possess their appropriate merits, and are admired by their respective customers.

For more particular information respecting the internal state of Southampton, we refer our readers to "Baker's and Skelton's Southampton Guides," and to "Cunningham's Register."

GENERAL INFORMATION.

Southampton contains three banks, all under very respectable firms. For physicians, it has been long distinguished; and happy is that person who, wanting medical assistance, obtains the care of the humane and skilful Dr. Mackie, who has been justly celebrated in a poem, entitled the "Physician," by kindred genius and philanthropy.

The post arrives daily from London, except on Monday, and there is likewise a cross-post from different places.

Coaches pass and repass daily from London, Portsmouth, Pool, Lymington, Bath, Bristol, and Salisbury: and to Oxford thrice a week; exclusive of other places, with which there is a frequent communication, by land as well as by water.

CAVALRY BARRACKS.

About half a mile from Bar-gate stand the barracks, a newly-erected building. The area is about two acres. The building is neat and plain, and capable of accommodating a troop of horse, with all the requisite conveniences and appendages.

THE POLYGON.

In this direction, and at a small distance, stands the

Polygon, which, if completed, would be the most beautiful assemblage of buildings in the kingdom. Only four houses are finished and inhabited, besides the hotel, which has been converted into two more private dwellings. The whole number was to have been twelve, with proper offices. Round it is a fine gravel road, to which company frequently resort for an airing, and to enjoy the beauty of the prospects.

WALKS AND RIDES ROUND SOUTHAMPTON.

So numerous are the seats, elegant and remarkable objects, and picturesque situations, round Southampton, that we must confine ourselves to a few, promiscuously selected.

NEW FOREST.

This extensive and beautiful tract contains more than 92000 superficial acres, its circumference being upwards of ninety miles. It is generally supposed to have been conveated into a forest by William the Conqueror, who, it is said, desecrated thirty-two churches, that he might enjoy his favourite pastime of hunting without interruption; but, it should be remembered, that churches were about four times more numerous at that æra than the present, and that William probably fixed on a spot already well-wooded, and thinly inhabited. The Conqueror seems to have undergone much obloquy on this account, and poets and puritans have united in his reprobation: Pope says,

The fields were ravish'd from the industrious swains,
From men their cities, and from gods their fanes;
The levell'd towns with weeds lie cover'd o'er;
The hollow winds through naked temples roar;
'Round broken columns clasping ivy twin'd;
O'er heaps of ruins stalk'd the stately hind;
The fox obscene to gaping tombs retires;
And savage howling fill the sacred choirs.

The misfortunes which attended the Conqueror's family on this spot, superstition has ascribed to the vengeance of heaven, for his profanation of its temples. His elder brother Richard, Richard his nephew, and William Rufus, his son and successor, all perished in the New Forest. The latter was accidentally slain by an arrow, from Sir Walter Tyrrell's bow, glancing against a tree, at a place called Canterton, near Stoney Cross, where the late Lord Delawar erected a triangular stone, with an inscription recording the circumstance of his death.

The New Forest is divided into nine bailiwicks, each under a master, keeper, and assistants. The superior officers are a lord warden, a lieutenant of the forest, a riding officer, bow-bearer, rangers, woodwards, verderors, high steward, &c.

This extensive tract is pleasantly diversified with hill and dale, heaths, and forest scenery. The oak, in particular, seems to delight in the soil; and, with better management, it would produce sufficient for half the navy of Great Britain.

The seasons for hunting are as follow: that of the hart and buck begins at St. John the Baptist, and ends on Holyrood day; of the hind and doe, begins at Holyrood and continues till Candlemas: of the fox, commences at Christmas and finishes at Lady-day; and of the hare, at Michaelmas and lasts till Candlemas. Forest shooting commences for grouse, or red game, the 12th of August; for heath-fowl, or black game, the 20th of August, and ends for both on the 10th of December.

Within the precincts of the New Forest and its environs, lie some handsome towns, populous villages, and various elegant seats.

Lyndhurst, near the centre of the forest, is a beautiful village, with roads branching from it in almost every direction. Here our ancient monarchs used to reside, while enjoying the pleasures of the chace. A large irregular mansion, called the King's House, built about the æra of Elizabeth, probably occupies the site where the hunting palace stood. It belongs now to the Duke of York, lord warden of the forest. The stabling is very extensive. His present Majesty visited this place in 1789; the Prince of Wales in 1791; and the Duke of Cumberland in 1802. A fox-hunt is established here, and many gentlemen have their hunting villas in the vicinity. The party of gentlemen who support the pack, assemble regularly in the month of March.

Mount Royal, so named by his Majesty when he visited this place in 1789, is situated on an elevated spot immediately contiguous to Lyndhurst, and the colonnade in front of the house commands one of the most magnificent views that can possibly be conceived. It is now called Northerwood by the present owner, though the change of name is neither honourable nor happy.

Cuffnels, the seat of the Right Hon. George Rose, esq. and member for Christ-church, is one of the most delightful residences in the kingdom. Nature has been liberal in its bounties to adorn it; but art has done more. Under the direction of Mrs. Rose, who appears to be as deeply skilled in landscape gardening as her husband is in finance, the principal improvements have taken place.

Foxlease, the residence of Isaac Pickering, esq. late of Sir Philip Jennings Clerke, bart. is a charming spot, though the situation is rather low. The house and grounds are advantageously viewed from Lyndhurst-green.

Brockenhurst, Watcombe, and Lymington,* have already been noticed; we proceed, therefore, to

Beaulieu, where, formerly, was an abbey of Cistercian monks. From the ruins, which are still considerable, it appears that the pile must have been very extensive. The refectory is entire, and has been converted into the parish church of Beaulieu. The prior's lodge is now a dwelling-house.

This monastery was founded by King John, in consequence, it is said, of a frightful dream. Un-

* See LYMINGTON.

principled as he was, superstition had the ascendancy over his mind.

Hythe is a neat and spacious village on Southampton river. Its marine and sylvan prospects are equally delightful. Ships frequently lie off this place.

Dibden stands opposite to Southampton, of which it commands the most charming views, as well as of the surrounding country.

Bury-house, the property of Sir Charles Mill, bart. with the appurtenant manor, is held by the singular tenure of presenting the king, whenever he enters the confines of the New Forest, a brace of milk-white greyhounds. A breed of these dogs is constantly preserved by the family, in readiness. His present majesty received this compliment in 1789.

ELING.

This pretty village lies at the head of Southampton river, and carries on a considerable trade in corn. It contains some very neat edifices, and here are docks for building and repairing ships. From the church-yard the prospect is very fine.

REDBRIDGE.

This large village, distant four miles from Southampton, lies nearly opposite to Eling. It had formerly a small abbey. It carries on some trade in coal, timber, and corn. Vessels of considerable size are built here.

GROVE-PLACE.

This is the seat of Mr. Jarratt, and stands about five miles from Southampton, on the Romsey-road, in a pleasant situation, with very picturesque views.

ROMSEY.

At the distance of seven miles from Southampton stands the market-town of Romsey, which is pretty large and well built. It was formerly famous for its monastery of Benedictine Nuns, founded by King Edgar. The only daughter of King Stephen was abbess of this nunnery, when she was carried off and married by Matthew Count of Alsace. After living ten years with him, and having two children, the terrors of the church overcame the force of duty and affection, and she was compelled to return and immure herself again in this place.

The church, which formerly belonged to the nunnery, is a noble edifice, built in the form of a cross, and arched with stone. It is a beautiful specimen of Saxon architecture, and contains several ancient monuments, which attract the notice of the curious.

In this town was born Sir William Petty, ancestor of the Marquis of Lansdown, and here he was interred, under a flat stone, with this brief memorial:

Here lies
Sir William Petty.

A beautiful monument to the memory of Frances Viscountess Palmerston, who died in child-bed, June 1, 1769, is as much admired for the virtues it commemorates, as for the skill of the sculptor. The inscription is too long to copy; but we cannot forbear inserting the following lines, written on the same melancholy subject, by the husband of this lady, the late Lord Palmerston. They have been given to different authors; and, though public fame was never the object of his lordship's regard, and now cannot avail him, it is but justice to his memory to restore to him what is undoubtedly his.

Whoe'er, like me, with trembling anguish brings
His heart's whole treasure to fair Bristol's springs;
Whoe'er, like me, to soothe distress and pain,
Shall court these salutary springs in vain;
Condemn'd like me, to hear the faint reply,
To mark the fading cheek, the sinking eye;
From the chill brow to wipe the damps of death,
And watch, in dumb despair, the short'ning breath;—
If chance should bring him to this artless line,
Let the sad mourner know his pangs were mine;

Ordained to lose the partner of my breast,
Whose virtue warm'd me, and whose beauty blessed;
Fram'd every tie that binds the heart to prove,
Her duty friendship, and her friendship love.
But yet, rememb'ring that the parting sigh
Appoints the just to slumber—not to die,
The starting tear I check'd; I kiss'd the rod;
And not to earth resign'd her—but to God.

In this church is a good organ; and what is deemed a singular curiosity, a fine apple-tree grows on the leads of the roof, and produces excellent fruit, though it must be very old.

BROADLANDS.

Half a mile from Romsey, towards Southampton, lies Broadlands, the seat of Lord Palmerston, descended from Sir William Temple. Both the exterior and interior of this splendid seat are finished in the highest stile of elegance. The gardens are tastefully laid out; and the park, through which the Test meanders, is well-wooded and finely varied. Over the Test, on the road to Salisbury, an elegant bridge has been lately built, of free stone, at the expence of the county, under the direction of Mr. Milne, the architect of Blackfriars-bridge.

HURSLEY.

At this pleasant village, which lies about eight miles from Southampton, on the road from Romsey to Winchester, is the seat of Sir William Heathcote, bart. formerly the property and occasional residence of Oliver Cromwell, and his son and successor Richard. The woods and shrubberies are extensive; the gardens handsomely disposed, and the park well stocked with deer. The house is a modern edifice; but a small part of the furniture is said to have belonged to the hypocritical protector.

CRANBURY.

The seat of Sir Nathaniel Holland, bart. better known as Nathaniel Dance, esq. one of our best painters, while painting was his profession, is one of the most delightful situations round Southampton, where beauties are so numerous, that it is difficult to select. It stands on the left, between Southampton and Winchester, and enjoys the most charming prospects of Southampton river and the Isle of Wight.

BELLEVUE.

This delightful seat stands within a mile of Southampton, on the road towards Winchester. It is a superb building within itself, but its scenery is so various and beautiful that no language can do it adequate justice. There are several fine buildings and commanding situations contiguous, but this eclipses them all.

BEVIS MOUNT.

Half a mile further, in the same direction, stands the agreeable seat of Edward Horne, esq. called Padwell, but more generally known by the name of Bevis* Mount. It lies on the banks of the Itchin, and was originally a vast pile of earth, rising in a conical form, supposed to have been an ancient fortification thrown up by the Saxons, to oppose the passage of the Danes. Below this mount the tide forms a fine bay, which is seen to great advantage from a summer-house. Lord Peterborough, the friend of Pope, once possessed this property, which he adorned with gardens, statues, walks, and plantations. The spot is equally romantic and pleasing.

PORTSWOOD-HOUSE.

This is a new and elegant edifice, lying on the Portsmouth road, about two miles from Southamp-

* Sir Bevis seems to have been the patron giant of Southampton. He was a Saxon knight of amazing strength and courage, and is reported to have resided here. His sword is still shewn in Arundel Castle.

ton. It was built by General Stibbert in 1776, and contains a good collection of paintings, by ancient and modern masters. The situation is commanding to an uncommon degree, and the accompaniments are all in the most enchanting and magnificent style.

ST. DIONYSIUS, OR DENNIS.

At a small distance from Portswood house, on the banks of the Itchin, stand the small remains of this ancient priory of canons of St. Austin, founded by Henry I. A farm-house occupies the scite, where may be seen some stone coffins, converted to troughs and other base purposes.

WOOD MILLS.

Higher up the Itchin are Wood Mills, the property of Mr. Taylor, who carries on by patent an extensive manufactory of ship-blocks, &c. for his majesty's dock-yards. The mechanism and facility with which the business is conducted is admirable. The spot forms a favourite aquatic excursion from Southampton, and in the passage, Bittern, the ancient Clausentum, may be seen to the best advantage.

SOUTH STONEHAM.

Four miles from Southampton, on the right of the Itchin, stands the mansion of South Stoneham, the seat of Mr. Bazalgette, in a pleasant but sequestered situation. The parish church is near the house.

NORTH STONEHAM.

This spacious edifice, which has been lately improved and enlarged, is situated about four miles from Southampton, to the right of the Winchester road. At the upper end of the park, which is extensive, is an elegant summer-house, which commands a profusion of the most captivating views.

In the church, adjoining to the mansion, which

belongs to the Flemings, is the beautiful monument of that illustrious naval officer, Lord Hawke, with an appropriate inscription, which justly says,

"The bravery of his soul was equal to the dangers he encountered; the curious intrepidity of his deliberations superior even to the conquests he obtained. The annals of his life compose a period of naval glory, unparallelled in later times; for whenever he sailed, victory attended him. A prince, unsolicited, conferred on him favours, which he disdained to ask."

In the same church, the antient family of Fleming have been interred for ages.

NORTHAM.

Two miles from Southampton, on the Itchin, nearly opposite to Bittern, lies Northam, an ancient dock-yard, where men of war have been built. The bridge, which has recently been erected over the Itchin, near this place, is one of the greatest improvements that has been produced in this neighbourhood.

CHESSEL, ARCHER-HOUSE, HOOK, &C.

So numerous are the elegant seats in the environs of Southampton, that it is impossible to particularise them. Chessel, the seat of Mr. Lance, stands on the east side of the Itchin: Archer-house, near Bellevue, belongs to Mr. Harrison, and is built on the ground lately belonging to the royal Southampton archers. Hook, near Hamble, is a very extensive and elegant building, on Southampton water, at no great distance from the channel, commanding almost boundless views of the New Forest and the Isle of Wight. It is the property and residence of Governor Hornsby.

MILLBROOK.

This delightful village lies about two miles from Southampton, on the road to Redbridge. It contains several genteel houses. Near it is Freemantle, the residence of Mr. Jarrett, and the beautiful cottage of James Amyatt, esq. late one of the representatives for Southampton.

NETLEY-ABBEY.

The picturesque and still beautiful ruins of Netley Abbey, formerly *Letley*, from *lætus locus*, as it is supposed, lie about six miles from Southampton by land, and four by water, on the gentle declivity of a hill, a small distance from Southampton river, anciently Tritenton. They are so surrounded by venerable woods, as scarcely to be discovered before they are approached; but, towards the river, there are some openings which, ever and anon, catch a glimpse of the passing sail.

The profusion of luxuriant ivy which covers the mouldering walls, the shrubs and trees which occupy the area of the church, where numerous dead repose, under fragments of elegant architecture and masses of ruins, the magnificence and extent of those parts which are still standing, compose a picture equally interesting and sublime. Such a scene reads many an impressive lesson on the vanity of human labours, and the uncertain hopes of fame, erected on such perishable foundations.

Now sunk, deserted, and with weeds o'ergrown,
　Yon prostrate walls their awful fate bewail;
Low on the ground their top-most spires are thrown,
　Once friendly marks, to guide the wand'ring sail.

The ivy now with rude luxuriance bends
　Its tangled foliage through the cloister'd space,
O'er the green window's mould'ring height ascends,
　And fondly clasps it with a last embrace.

While the self-planted oak, within confin'd
　(Auxiliar to the tempest's wild uproar)
Its giant branches fluctuate to the wind,
　And rend the wall whose aid it courts no more.

KEATE'S ELEGY.

Netley is generally supposed to have been founded by Henry III, about the year 1239, for monks of the Cistercian order, and dedicated to the Virgin Mary and St. Edward. Roger de Clare, and John de Warrenne, earl of Surry, were afterwards its principal benefactors. Little, indeed, is known of its history, and it is probably more noticed in its ruins than it was in all its original splendour.

At the dissolution, it consisted of an abbot and twelve monks, whose possessions, according to Dugdale, were valued at 100*l.* 12*s.* 8*d.* and according to Speed, at 160*l.* 2*s.* 9*d.*

The site was granted to Sir William Paulet by Henry VIII. About the middle of the sixteenth century, it was the seat of one of the earls of Hertford, and since that period we find it in the possession of an earl of Huntingdon, who converted part of the chapel into a kitchen and other offices, reserving the eastern end for a place of worship.

It appears that this nobleman, or, as some say, sir Bartlett Lucy, agreed with a Mr. Taylor, of Southampton, for the purchase of so much of the materials as he could carry away within a limited time: a contract which was fatal to Mr. Taylor.

The circumstances which led to Mr. Taylor's catastrophe are variously related; but the following are the most generally believed. After he had engaged for the demolition of this venerable place, he dreamed one night, that the arch key-stone of one of the windows fell, and fractured his skull.—Strongly impressed with this dream, he communicated its purport to some of his friends, who advised him to avoid being personally concerned in the business; but in his eagerness to make an advantage of his bargain, hastily tearing down some boards, a stone fell on his head. The fracture was not thought to be mortal at first, but the surgeon's instrument slipping in the operation of extracting a splinter, entered the brain, and caused immediate death. The family of this Mr. Taylor still live in Southampton,

Another dreamer is said to have been more fortunate. A farmer's labourer having been repeatedly informed, in his sleep, of money being concealed in a certain part of the ruins, at length searched for it, and found a chest, containing coins to a considerable amount.

Every visitor of Southampton makes an excursion to Netley, and generally by water. The Fountain Court, a large area with some trees in it, and having its walls clamped with ivy, first receives us. On the right of this court is an apartment, which was probably the refectory; and, adjoining to it, are the pantry and kitchen. The latter is a large vaulted room with a curious fire-place; opposite to which a subterraneous passage is pointed out, supposed to lead to the neighbouring fort, one of those erected by Henry VIII. which has suffered less from time than the abbey.

Returning through the refectory, visit the Chapter-house; and, passing two smaller rooms, enter the abbey-church by the cross aisle. Part of the church still remains; its beautiful eastern window is universally admired; and, till within a few years, some portions of the fine arched ceiling were standing.

> Within the shelter'd centre of the aisle,
> Beneath the ash, whose growth romantic spreads
> Its foliage, trembling o'er the funeral pile,
> And all around a deeper darkness sheds;
> While through yon arch, where the thick ivy twines,
> Bright on the silver'd tower the moon-beam shines,
> And the grey cloister's roofless length illumes,
> Upon the mossy stone I lie reclin'd,
> And to a visionary world resign'd,
> Call the pale spectres forth from the forgotten tombs.
>
> SOTHEBY'S NETLEY ABBEY.

The ancient city of Winchester, the Saxon metropolis, and the place where many of the kings of that line are buried, lies within twelve miles of Southampton, or within a morning ride. Its cathedral and other antiquities are well worth visiting. Here, too, is the shell of the noble palace begun by Charles II. generally used as barracks in time of peace, or as a prison for captives in time of war. Its situation is extremely commanding; and, had the pile been completed, it would have been worthy the residence of the most powerful kings on earth.

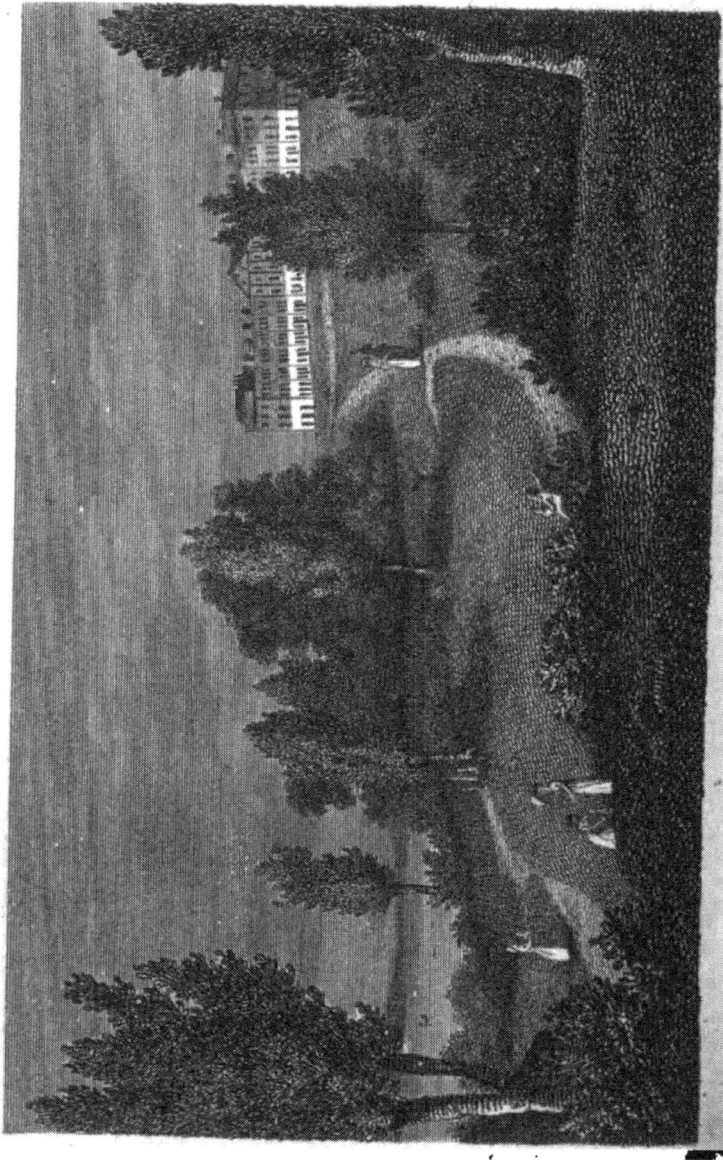

View of Terrace at Southend.

SOUTHEND.

SOUTHEND, in Essex, became noticed as a watering-place about fifteen years ago. It is eligibly situated on the slope of a well-cultivated and a well-wooded hill, about forty-three miles from London, and three from Rochford, and lies at the mouth of the Thames, nearly opposite to Sheerness.

The soil is sandy and the shore flat, and so shallow, that at low water a stranger would suppose that the sea had totally abandoned the place. The air is esteemed very dry and salubrious, and the water, notwithstanding its mixture with the Thames, is clear, and sufficiently salt. Besides the machines, which are neat and commodious, here are two warm baths.

The terrace, which is commonly called New Southend, being built on a considerable eminence, gives the houses a stately and elegant appearance, especially from the Thames; the houses run in a long line, and are handsomely finished with pilasters and cornices of stone. They command a most delightful and extensive view of the sea, the Nore, the Medway, Sheerness, and of the shipping bound to, or returning from, the emporium of the world.

New Southend remained nearly stationary some years, owing to the failure of the first proprietors of the Terrace and adjacent buildings. In the year 1800, however, the property being sold by auction, passed into the hands of James Heygate, esq. and John Thomas Hope, esq. In addition to these gentlemen, Sir Thomas Wilson, Lady Langham, and other families, possess houses on the Terrace, and reside at this village a considerable part of the year. The number of summer visitants has recently encreased rapidly, and among them have been personages of the first distinction, particularly her Royal Highness the Princess of Wales.

The Assembly-room is handsomely finished, but is not regularly filled at any stated periods. Sometimes, however, the company is pretty numerous, and they are mostly of the superior ranks of society; the lower orders of the community not having as yet intruded themselves into Southend, as into many other places of this description.

A Theatre was erected here in 1804. It is very well attended, and is under the management of Mr. Trotter, who conducts the dramatic amusements in a respectable and satisfactory manner.

The Library is an elegant building, somewhat in the gothic stile, and is beautifully situated on the brow of the hill, between what are called the old and new town.

The Hotel, which is situated at the eastern extremity of the Terrace, is extremely spacious and convenient, nor are the Ship Tavern, and Hope Inn, wanting in adequate accommodations.

There is also a chapel, for the use of dissenters, at this place.

The country round Southend is rich and populous, and agriculture is carried on with assiduity and success. The white-fronted dwellings of the yeomanry and peasants, add considerably to the picturesque effect of the landscape. There is, in short, every appearance of comfort and content, even among the lowest classes, which cannot but afford a sweet sensation to every benevolent mind, so apt to be pained by sights of misery at places of fashionable resort.

A daily coach sets out for Southend from the Bull Inn, Aldgate; also a vessel for the conveyance of passengers and luggage leaves Wheeler's Wharf, St. Catherine's, for this place once a week.

Not far from Southend, a stone is placed to mark the jurisdiction of the Lord Mayor of London.

RIDES AND WALKS ROUND SOUTHEND.

The adjacent country is well wooded, and abounds with game, a circumstance which must render this place a pleasant residence in the season for sporting gentlemen. The roads are excellent, which is the more extraordinary, as there is only one turnpike in the neighbourhood for many miles.

LEIGH.

Leigh is a small port-town, famous for its oyster fishing, and lying near Southend, furnishes an opportunity of being supplied with that delicate article of food.

This fishing is so precarious, that individuals can seldom afford to risk engaging in it. It is, therefore, usually carried on by a company, who annually proceed to Cancalle Bay, on the coast of France, from whence they bring the young brood of the oyster in a jelly-like form, not larger than a shilling, and laying them on the sands or grounds near the town, from some peculiar quality in the soil, in about three months they acquire their full growth and consistence. The nature of this shore, and its adaptation for feeding oysters, were accidentally discovered by a person of the name of Outing, about 1700, who, taking a lease of this district, soon made a fortune.

Camden calls this a pretty little town, stocked with lusty seamen. The church is pleasantly situate on the top of a hill, and is dedicated to St. Clement, one of the first bishops of Rome, who suffered martyrdom, as is said, by having an anchor tied to his neck, and then thrown into the sea.

CANVEY-ISLAND.

This spot, which deserves notice as having been in a manner wrested from the watery element, is about five miles long and two broad. The land being subject to be overflowed, the proprietors agreed to give one third of it in fee simple to a Dutchman, skilled in making dykes, on condition of his securing it from the tide. He effected much; but it is still subject to inundations at high floods. One which happened in 1735 destroyed half the cattle on the island.

Canvey is formed by the channel which runs from Leigh up to South Bamfleet, and continues to Old Haven, where it again meets the Thames.

HADLEIGH-CASTLE.

This castle stands at a small distance westward of Leigh. It was built by Hubert de Burgh, earl of Kent, in the reign of Henry III. and its existing ruins show its original grandeur. In process of time it came to Thomas of Woodstock, who is said to have been smothered with pillows at Calais, in 1397.

Only three or four lofty towers remain to attest its ancient magnificence. The site is almost overgrown with bushes; but, being situated on the brow of a steep hill, it commands a delightful prospect across the Thames into Kent.

ROCHFORD.

This ancient town is distant about three miles from Southend, and forty from London; it is seated on a small stream which falls into the Crowch, in a damp and unhealthy situation.

On an eminence near this town, called King's-hill, the lord of the manor of Rayleigh, a place about seven miles off, holds a court at midnight on the first Wednesday after Michaelmas, which is kept till cock-crowing. This is called Lawless-court. The steward and suitors are obliged to whisper to each other, and are not allowed either fire or candle. A piece of coal supplies the place of pen and ink; and, he who owes service to the court and fails in his attendance, forfeits double his rent, for every hour's absence. It is said, that this attendance was originally imposed on the tenants, as a punishment for their having met, at this place, in a conspiracy against their lord.

PRITTLEWELL.

This large village, which lies at a small distance from Southend, was formerly famous for a priory, founded by Robert de Essex, or Fitz Swale, for monks of the Cluniac order. It was dedicated to the Virgin Mary, and endowed with the tithes of several parishes.

SWANSEA.

Glamorgan, in which Swansea lies, is a maritime county of South Wales, enjoying, except in the northern part, a mild and salubrious air. It produces wood, corn, mines of coal and iron, and verifies the panegyric of its native bard, who says,

Glamorgan boast thy sky serene;
Thy health-inspiring gales;
Thy sunny plains luxuriant green;
Thy graceful mountain's airy scene;
Thy wild romantic vales.

The greatest part of the sea-coast forms a semicircular sweep; but towards Swansea, its principal port, it becomes deeply indented, and projecting into a narrow beak, between the open channel on the one hand, and an arm, winding round to the Caermarthenshire coast on the other.

SITUATION AND GOVERNMENT, &c.

Swansea, a pleasant well-built town on the river Towy, and a fashionable watering-place, distant about 206 miles from London, stands near the centre of a beautiful bay, on an angle between two hills, which shelter it from the cold winds, and allow it an opening to the south. It lies mid-way between Bristol and Tenby, and has of late received several considerable improvements.

Being built on a semicircular rising bank, near the mouth of the Towy, the towns makes a very handsome appearance from the road approaching to it; and, in particular, a fine bird's-eye view may be seen from the round tower of the castle, or Kilvey-hill, whence the whole is brought into a distinct and beautiful perspective, forming an irregular oblong, nearly a mile and a half in length, charmingly intersected by the meanders of the river, and varied with the shipping and small craft that frequent the harbour.

Swansea is a borough-town, governed by a portreve, recorder, twelve aldermen, two common attornies or chamberlains, and an unlimited number of burgesses. Together with the six other contributary boroughs, it returns a member to parliament; and, on account of its elegance, opulence, population, and extent, justly ranks as the first town in the county.

BUILDINGS AND ACCOMMODATIONS.

The Burrows, as they are called, contain many pleasant lodging-houses. Here, likewise, is an excellent warm sea-water bath, and a chapel for the Whitfieldian methodists.

Wind-street is handsome and well paved, at one end of which is the Look-out, the Custom-house, one of the Circulating Libraries, the Post-office, and the Glamorgan Bank.

The Mackworth Arms is a good house of accommodation. At some distance is the market-place, for corn, fish, and vegetables. On the left is Butter-street, or rather St. Mary's, where the butchers and country people expose their respective articles for sale; on the right are the remains of the old castle, now converted into a goal and workhouse.

This castle, which must have been an extensive pile, was burnt by Griffin Prince of South Wales, soon after its erection, which was about the year 1113.

Near the castle is the old mansion of the lords of the manor, built round a quadrangle; and, joining the former fabric, is a modern-built town-hall, near which is the new market, erected in 1774, where petty articles of common necessity are sold on Wednesdays.

Worcester-place consists of a range of neat houses, all the property of one person, and so called in honour of the Marquis of Worcester.

Between the market and the Higher Town, is Castle Bailey-street, divided in the middle by a strait line of stones, ranged longitudinally, and so denominated, because that part next the castle secures the prisoner for debt from molestation, provided he does not exceed the bounds prescribed.

Beyond this is the High-street, or Upper Town, running nearly a mile in length, and containing many excellent houses. Here stands the Ivy-bush Tavern, which is well adapted for the reception of company. Near this is a dissenting meeting-house, and far up is the church of St. John's, now almost dilapidated.

Mount Pleasant is a charming situation, and the houses are frequently inhabited by persons of fashion. Bellevue, the residence of Cuthbert Johnson, esq. and Heathfield-lodge, the elegant seat of sir Gabriel Powell, with some others in this quarter, command the most picturesque scenery.

Goat-street, likewise, contains many commodious houses. Here stands the Grammar-school, endowed by Hugh Lord Bishop of Waterford and Lismore. Near it is a chapel for the numerous disciples of the late John Wesley; and, in a ruinous house, at the corner of the street, that celebrated character Richard Nash, esq. who so many years ruled the fashionable world at Bath, was born.

BATHS, &C.

Half a mile from the town, on the beach, stands the bathing-house, excellently adapted for its destination; and, from the windows of the appurtenant ball-room, there is a fine view of the bay, and the coast of Devonshire.

The terms and regulations are: Board and Lodging, 1*l.* 11*s.* 6*d.* per week; ditto, for servants, 1*l.* 1*s.*; private parlour, 10*s.* 6*d.* per week; dogs, 2*s.* per week; bathing, an hour before or after high water, 1*s.* each time.

Jordan's warm sea-water baths are situate on the Burrows. Bathing, each time 3*s.* in summer; and 3*s.* 6*d.* in the winter half-year.

Haynes's cold and hot sea-water baths stand near the pottery. The terms are as follow: Cold-bath, with a fire in the dressing-room, 1*s.* 3*d.*; without fire, 1*s.*; guide, 6*d.* Hot bath, with a fire in dressing-room. 3*s.*; without fire, 2*s.* 9*d.*; guide, 6*d.* Here, also, are pumps for partial bathing, and a shower-bath. In a word, Swansea possesses every accommodation for using the marine fluid with effect. The bay is universally allowed to be singularly beautiful, and the shore is very commodious for bathing.

FERRY.

To the ferry, where persons, cattle, and goods, are passed over on moderate terms, each tenement in the parish of Swansea, and in the lower division of Llansamlet, and every housekeeper in the township of Swansea, is chargeable with 4*d.* a-year; and in the higher division of Llansamlet, with 2*d.* a-year. Ferry-side house furnishes good entertainment to visitors, and a few lodgings are let here during the season.

STRAND.

On the Strand, which is of considerable length, is a commodious quay, where many vessels of considerable burthens are annually built. Along this and the Burrows, is a pleasant promenade, furnishing some delightful scenery.

TRADE.

The commerce of Swansea arises chiefly from the various mines of coal and culm in the vicinity, and this has been rapidly increasing of late years. In 1791, an act of parliament was obtained, for repairing enlarging, and preserving the harbour, with the power of borrowing 12,000*l.* and of levying certain rates per ton, on all shipping trading to the port. The provisions of this act being duly carried into execution, under trustees of the first respectability, improvements are rapidly carrying on; and such regulations are established as are most likely to promote and confirm the rising prosperity of the town and port. Upwards of 2,500 vessels annually enter or leave the harbour.

CHURCH.

The church, dedicated to St. Mary, is modern and well built; consisting of a middle and two side aisles seventy-two feet long, by fifty-four wide. The whole is neatly paved, and contains a gallery and an organ. At the east end is a plain tower, with six bells. There are several monuments in this church, but none remarkable.

CIRCULATING LIBRARIES, BILLIARD-TABLES, &c. &c.

Swansea, in common with other places of public resort, has its rival Libraries, and both are filled with a good assortment of the usual articles. Though the scholar would be disappointed, those who seek only for amusement, will be sufficiently gratified.

At Oakey's Circulating Library, in Wind-street, the terms of the circulating books are,

For a Year	£1	0	0
a Quarter	0	10	6
a Month	0	6	0

Terms of the Reading-room.

Newspapers & Periodical Publications, by Subscription.

For a Year	£1	1	0
a Half-year	0	10	6
a Quarter	0	6	0
a Month	0	2	6

At Evans's Circulating Library, in the same street, the terms are considerably lower.

For yearly Subscribers	£0	16	0
Half-yearly	0	8	6
Quarterly	0	4	6
Monthly	0	2	0
Single volume	0	0	3

At the George, in Wind-street, are a good and well-frequented Ball-court, and Billiard-table; and at the Fountain, and Red Lion, in the Strand, are other billiard-tables.

COACHES AND PACKETS.

A mail-coach from London arrives every morning at Swansea, through Bristol, about five o'clock; and from Milford about eight every evening, from whence it sets out immediately for London. There are also some cross-posts.

Coasting vessels frequently sail from London, Bristol, Gloucester, and various parts of the coasts of Cornwall, Devon, and Somerset.

Packets regularly sail to Dublin, Waterford, and Cork; and constantly twice a week, and sometimes thrice, to Ilfracombe. Fares for passengers to the latter place, 10*s.* 6*d.* each.

POPULATION.

According to the enumeration of inhabitants, taken in 1801, Swansea was found to contain 2872 males, and 3959 females: in all, 6831.

CAMBRIAN POTTERY.

This useful establishment, conducted by Mr. Haynes, on the Strand, is well worthy the attention of those who have never had an opportunity of seeing this kind of manufacture.

The clay used here is brought from various parts of England; and, being afterwards mixed in water, with finely-powdered flint, is passed through sieves, till all the coarser particles are excluded. It is then exposed to heat, after which, the air and water being evaporated by drying and beating, the clay becomes fit for working.

A piece of it being stuck on a circular board, with an horizontal rotation, a rude vessel is almost instantly formed by the artist. Coloring, glazing, painting, stamping, drying, and baking, follow in progressive order; and many elegant articles, which employ numerous hands, are produced from substances of comparatively little value, to the equal benefit of the proprietor and the public.

WALKS AND RIDES ROUND SWANSEA.

In the immediate vicinity of Swansea, are several pleasant walks and objects, which we shall casually notice, before we take a few more distant excursions.

St. Helen's, the seat of Capt. Jones, lies about a mile to the westward; and a mile further is Marino, a curious octagonal building, belonging to Edward King, esq.; near this is Veranda; and, at no great distance, is Sketty-lodge, the residence of Mr. Phillips, which, being situated on an eminence, commands the whole of Swansea-bay.

Across the river is Black-hill, Cline-wood, and the Woodlands, a house in the gothic stile, belonging to Colonel Ward. Near the beach stands Lilliput-hall; which, from the smallness of its dimensions, not ill deserves the title; but its accompaniments are so beautiful, that the building is overlooked in the estimate which is formed of the place.

OYSTERMOUTH CASTLE AND VILLAGE.

On leaving the brow of an eminence near the beach, surrounded by broken cliffs of lime-stone, stand the majestic ruins of Oystermouth-castle, said to have been built by Henry Earl of Warwick; it now appertains to the Duke of Beaufort. The entrance to the castle is at the south end, which projects to break the square; and on a level with the wall, on the east side is the keep, from whence the prospect is extremely fine. From what remains of this castle, it is evident it must have contained many spacious apartments, and that it was once a place of great strength.

A little further on is Oystermouth church, a very picturesque object from many situations, as well as the village of the same name, which lying along the bottom of a high lime-stone rock, loses all sight of the sun for upwards of three months in the year. In this vicinity, on the head of a peninsula, is erected a light-house, a building much admired, and frequently visited by the company from Swansea.

Contiguous to this, and along the coast, is some fine rocky scenery, particularly in the beautiful bay of Caswell.

PENNARTH-CASTLE.

About six miles from Swansea, are the romantic ruins of Pennarth-castle; the access to which is extremely difficult, from the deep loose sand-banks that surround it. The neighbouring peasantry believe it was raised in one night, by enchantment, and fancy it is still the residence of fairies.

ARTHUR'S STONE.

On the north-west point of Cevin-Brin, one of the highest mountains in South Wales, is a vast stone of alabaster, twenty tons weight, supported by six or seven others, about four feet high, set circularly. This stupendous Cromlech is called Arthur's Stone, from the hero who is supposed to have erected it.

THE CANAL.

By the side of the canal, which extends from Swansea pottery to Hen-noyadd, in Brecon, are many capital objects, and the walk along it is very pleasant. There are no fewer than 36 locks in the space of sixteen miles, and several aqueducts. Adjoining, are large smelting copper-works, an iron forge, tin and brass works, a fine copper rolling-mill, iron furnaces, a foundery, and a most stupendous steam-engine, at Llandwr, which throws up, from a vast depth, 100 gallons of water every stroke, or twelve times a minute, making 78,000 gallons in an hour.

NEATH.

The town of Neath, the Nidum of Antoninus, is seated at the bottom of a valley, on the banks of the river Nedd. The streets are irregular and narrow, and the houses generally ill-built, while the air is loaded with the smoke of the copper-works in the vicinity. This circumstance must, of necessity, render the place unwholesome; yet, its population amounts to between 2 and 3000 souls, and its commerce is considerable. A few ruins of its old castle, probably built by Richard de Greenfield, a Norman, still remain.

Neath Abbey, about half a mile west of the town, is a very picturesque object. The mouldering remains, which looks so attractive at a distance, are tenanted by the miserable families of the workmen, employed at the neighbouring copper smelting-houses. In this vicinity is an inexhaustible store of coals.

On an eminence near Neath stands Gnoll castle, an elegant seat most delightfully situated, built by the late Sir Herbert Mackworth, and now in the possession of Mr. Leigh.

CASCADE OF MELLINCOURT.

Five miles from Neith, is the celebrated cascade of Mellincourt, where the river Clydaugh precipitates itself from the height of eighty feet.

BRITTON-FERRY.

Britton-Ferry, the elegant mansion of Lord Vernon, abounds in the most captivating scenery. The situation of the house is pleasingly sequestered, being embosomed in the most luxuriant foliage, contrasted with grey broken rocks, agreeably intermixed. The lover of nature will be enchanted with this spot, and the artist will find it to comprise a school of landscape in itself.

MARGAM PARK.

Margam Park is of considerable extent, and excellently stocked. It is completely sheltered from the north, by a hill of great height and length. The green-house is unquestionably the largest in the kingdom, measuring 129 yards by twenty-seven. It was originally built for the reception of a fine collection of orange and lemon-trees, which was wrecked on the coast.

At each end of this noble green-house is an apartment containing models of old buildings, ancient marbles and statues, well worth a careful inspection.

To those who are inclined to take more distant excursions from Swansea, we would recommend a visit to Clare Cennin Castle, four miles south-east of Llandillo, an undoubted ancient British erection; to St. Donat's Castle, situated on a rock, impending the shore, five miles south-west of Cowbridge; to the Pont-y-Prydd, or New Bridge, a stupendous arch thrown across the river Taaf, the work of William Edwards, a common mason; to Llandaff, the ancient see of a bishop; to Caerphilly Castle, remarkable for its leaning tower, which projects eleven feet over its base; and to the beautiful town and castle of Cardiff.

Few counties can be more interesting to the antiquary and the naturalist * than Glamorganshire; but, possessing, as it does, numerous local advantages, it seems more pleasant to the occasional visitor, than the constant resident. The volumes of smoke continually arising from the numerous and extensive works that are established here, render many parts unpleasant, if not insalubrious, even to those who live at some distance, while the sickly looks, and the dissipated habits of the workmen, too feelingly prove that mines and founderies are equally the bane of health and morals.

* The botanist, in particular, will find a rich harvest of rare plants along the shores, and among the hills of this district.

TEIGNMOUTH *and* SHALDON.

TEIGNMOUTH, in Devonshire, derives its name from its situation at the mouth of the Teign, by whose estuary it is separated from Shaldon, another bathing-place of modern date, which will be noticed in the sequel.

SITUATION AND HISTORY.

Teignmouth, distant 187 miles from London, and 14 from Exeter, is noticed in the chronicles of ancient times. It stands at the efflux of the Teign, which romantic river rises on the forest of Dartmoor. The mouth here is nearly choaked up with sand, which renders it inaccessible for any but small vessels; though this place had once a good trade with Newfoundland and America. Here the Danes landed about the year 800, and having defeated the natives, spread their ravages into the interior of the country. In latter times it was plundered and partly burnt by the French; but rose with superior beauty from the ashes. As a memorial of this disaster, one of the streets has the name of French-street. It is divided into two parishes, East and West Teignmouth, separated from each other by a rivulet called the Tame. From the north and north-east winds it is sheltered by rising hills, near the foot of which stands the pleasant village of Shaldon in front, and the wide expanse of ocean on the east. The two parishes, east and west, contain together about 1850 inhabitants.

WEST TEIGNMOUTH.

West Teignmouth formerly had, by charter, a market on Sundays, which continued to the time of Henry III. when this irreligious practice was put down. There is now a market every Saturday for poultry, butcher's meat, fish of various kinds, butter, vegetables, and fruit. By an excellent local regulation, the inhabitants are allowed to supply themselves with fish, before any is sold to the dealers. Salmon, salmon-peel, sea-trout, whiting, mackarel, and other kinds of choice fish, are caught here in abundance.

There are several good houses here: the principal of which are Teignmouth-house, the residence of Mr. Baring, and Bitton, the seat of Mr. Praed, and the cottage of Mrs. Boscawen.

The church at West Teignmouth, standing near the centre of the town, is built in the form of a cross: its roof is curiously supported by the ramifications of a wooden pillar, running up the middle. Here are several neat monuments: and the whole is commodiously fitted up. This church is appendant on the living of Bishop's Teignton.

EAST TEIGNMOUTH.

This is now the grand resort of company, as furnishing the best lodgings, which may be hired, furnished or unfurnished, at the option of the renter.

The Public Rooms form a neat brick building, containing apartments for tea, coffee, assembly, and billiards. A ball is held every fortnight or three weeks, and sometimes oftener, according to the wishes of the company.

The theatre, built on a spot of ground given by lord Courtenay, is fully adequate to the purpose for which it is intended.

The bathing-machines are sufficiently commodious. The beach, composed of smooth sands, with occasional layers of small pebbles, gradually slopes to the sea, which is generally clear and clean, and sheltered from all except the east winds.

East Teignmouth church stands near the beach. It is a venerable pile, and bears marks of Saxon, or at least early Norman, architecture, as may be inferred from the round tower. Connected with the square one, the narrow windows with semicircular arches, and the corbels, or heads of men and animals, placed as ornamental supports to the parapet, attract the eye of the passenger. It is an appendage to the living of Dawlish, as West Teignmouth is to Bishop's Teignton. These two incumbents nominate the minister, who serves the parishes alternately.

TRADE.

The prosperity of Teignmouth, in a great measure, depends on its summer visitors. Its chief commerce consists in the exportation of pipe-clay to Bristol, Staffordshire, Liverpool, and other places. Some vessels are however built here.

INNS, &c.

There are two inns, the Globe and Hubbard's hotel. From the Globe, a coach goes and returns the same day, thrice a week, to Exeter. The hotel possesses good accommodations; and, from the billiard-room belonging to it, there is a most delightful and extensive view up the river, with all its picturesque and moving scenery.

PROMENADES.

The "Walk," as it is called, by eminence, leads from the Rooms towards the south, over a low flat between hills, called the Den, a track of fine sand, interspersed with patches of grass, which in dry weather assume a similar hue. For the accommodation of walkers, seats are placed in the most favourable situations for enjoying views of the sea, the cliffs, the range of the coast, and many interesting objects.

Among the scenes which will attract the attention of strangers, sein-drawing may be particularized. It is performed by women, in appropriate dresses, and the picture of hope, with the shade of disappointment, which they exhibit as the centre of the net approaches the shore, while they expect a full or empty haul, would furnish an excellent subject for the pencil. The whole shore, indeed, presents an animated and busy scene.

Another walk leads to the westward of the town, by the grove near Britton and the banks of the river, which at the recession of the tide, admits of a return on the sands.

From East Teignmouth church, a third road, much frequented, leads towards Dawlish under the cliffs, where the contemplative will delight to stray,

> And list, with pleasing dread, to the deep roar
> Of the wide weltering waves.

From these cliffs, and the hill in general, which backs the town, are many charming views of land and water.

SHALDON.

By a ferry pass the Teign to Shaldon, which lies adjacent to a promontory called the Ness. It contains some new-built lodging-houses, and is much admired as a summer residence, by those who love to blend with general retirement an occasional intercourse with the busy world. In fact, it is a charming village; and, from its lying so near Teignmouth, visitors may mix when they please with the society, and join the amusements of that place.

Shaldon is the property of lord Clifford, and lies partly in two parishes; St. Nicholas, and Stoke, in Teign Head. In the environs are some agreeable walks, but that upon the beach is most frequented, under the lofty aspiring Ness, which is of itself a sublime object. It is six miles east from Abbott's Newton.

RIDES FROM TEIGNMOUTH AND SHALDON.

The contiguity of these two places renders the rides of the one in general equally convenient for the other. For an airing, Haldon, four miles and a half south-west by south from Exeter, and its vicinity, is much used, and parties are frequently formed to visit the same places as were indicated in the rides from Dawlish. The more appropriate excursions are to

LINDRIDGE.

This capital mansion, the property of the Rev. John Templar, stands on a rich lawn, beautifully wooded, in the parish of Bishop's Teignton. The building is less extensive than formerly, when it was said to have occupied an acre of ground. The apartments are decorated with valuable paintings by Vandervelde, Vanbloom, and other eminent artists. A room, preserved in the original stile in which the mansion was fitted up, will give some idea of the splendour of its ancient possessors. The picturesque beauty of the grounds is uncommonly fine.

UGBROOK.

Ugbrook Park, the seat of lord Clifford, baron of Chudleigh, is reckoned one of the most charming spots in Devon. The approach is by a fine avenue of venerable trees; the grounds are delightfully varied, and in the words of the poet, who has made it the subject of his muse, we may observe, that,

> ———————— Collected here,
> As in one point, all Nature's charms appear.

This place must be seen; for it cannot be described with sufficient effect.

CHUDLEIGH.

Through this small but neat market-town, which is about seven miles from Teignmouth, runs the road from Exeter to Plymouth. In the vicinity, the bishops of Exeter had once a magnificent palace, the remains of which are still visible. The manor now belongs to lord Clifford.

About half a mile from the town, on the barton of Lowell, is Chudleigh-rock, according to Mr. Polwhele, "one of the most striking inland rocks in the island." Viewed from the west, it is a bold and beautiful perpendicular rock, apparently one solid mass of marble. From the south-east, a hollow opens to the view, with a stream rushing impetuously at the bottom of it, and here and there checked in its progress by a great quantity of rude stones scattered around. And the scenery is, in summer, rendered more attractive by a luxuriant wood, that seems proudly to bear forward its burthen of variegated foliage, on the opposite side. About midway, down the cliff, is a large cavern, with various intricate windings, which vulgar superstition assigns as the abode of fairies.

DREW-STEIGNTON.

This parish is remarkable for its romantic beauties and curiosities. On a farm called Shilstone, is the only Cromlech in this county. The covering stone, or quoit, hath three supporters; it rests on the pointed tops of the southern and western ones, but that on the north side supports it on its inner inclining surface. This latter supporter is seven feet high, and the dimensions of the quoit are each way about fourteen feet. But the most surprising object here is the rocking or logan-stone, which is a stupendous block of granite, resting at its base on a rising point of another mass, deep-grounded in the channel of the river Teign. The banks of this river are peculiarly attractive. The wildness of wood and rock, now washed by the Teign, now starting from the sides of the hills, seems the discriminating feature. South of the Cromlech, at a little distance, is a curious *logan*, or rocking-stone. It is in the midst of the Teign, and "is poised," says Polwhele, "upon another mass of stone, which is deep grounded in the bed of the river." It is in length about eighteen feet, west and east, and at the highest end, to the west, it is ten feet in height. It may be easily rocked with one hand; but its quantity of motion does not exceed one inch.

The surrounding scenery is singularly grand and

inviting. The hill of Piddle Down rises majestically high, and is encompassed by luxuriant trees of a rich and variegated foliage.

KING'S TEIGNTON.

This village, which used to be infested with agues, is become, by draining the marshes, pretty healthy. The church, with its grove of tall elms, has a good effect. It contains a tomb with this singular inscription:

Richardus Adlam, hujus Ecclesiæ
Vicarius, obiit Feb. 10th, 1670.
Apostrophe ad Mortem:

Damn'd tyrant! can't profaner blood suffice?
Must priests that offer be the sacrifice?
Go tell the genii that in Hades lye
Thy triumphs o'er this sacred Calvary;
'Till some just Nemesis avenge our cause,
And force this kill-priest to revere good laws!

HACCOMBE.

This mansion belongs to the family of the Carews, to whom it descended from its ancient lords, *de Haccombe*. Haccombe is said to be the smallest parish in England, containing only two dwellings, the mansion-house and the parsonage. It enjoys extraordinary privileges. It is not included in any hundred: no officer, civil or military, had a right to take cognizance of any proceedings in this parish; and, it was exempted from all duties and taxes, in consequence of some noble exploits performed by the Carews. In the chapel, a very picturesque object, are some curious monuments of the Haccombe and Carew families; and, on the southern door, are the fragments of four horse-shoes, belonging to a horse which is said to have swam with one of the Carews on his back, a great way into the sea, and back again, by which a considerable wager was won.

MAMHEAD.

The delightful seat of Wilmot, lord Lisburne, will afford considerable gratification to every visitor. It formerly was the property of the Balles, the last of whom adorned it with beautiful and extensive plantations. At the same time he fell into the old error of torturing nature, by raising gardens with terraces, and making ponds and fountains on the sides of hills. All this, however, was removed by the succeeding noble proprietor, who restored the ground to its pristine natural beauty, and Mamhead now appears as one extensive inclosure, with various prospects of sea, river, and the country. Towards Haldon, the most beautiful plantations of firs and forest trees in Devonshire, are crowned by a noble obelisk, which stands on Mamhead point, and consists of Portland stone, about 100 feet in height. In front of the house we cannot but admire the easy swell of the lawn, whose smooth verdure is relieved by groupes of trees and shrubs; whilst, at one extremity, the eye is attracted by General Vaughan's picturesque cottage, and a little beyond these grounds, by a landscape, which no scenery in this country exceeds in richness. On this side the Exe, are to be seen the ancient castle and possessions of Courtenay, with the villages of Kenton and Starcross; on the other side, Exmouth and Lympstone, with the country stretching away to the Somersetshire and Dorsetshire hills. In the mean time the river, and the sea, in full prospect, give a finishing touch to the whole, and renders it a picture of enchanting sublimity.

FORD.

At the foot of Milber Down stands Ford, built in the reign of James I. by Sir Richard Reynell. It was honoured with a visit by Charles I. who one day after dinner conferred the honour of knighthood on two brothers of that family. Here also William III.

took up his night's lodging, after landing in Torbay. The estate now belongs to the Courtenays, to whom it came by marriage. The house stands on a lawn, retired from the road, and opposite to it is a deer-park.

TOTNESS.

Near Totness the vestiges of a Roman road are still to be traced. This was once a walled town, with four gates, but only one of them is now standing. The ruins of the castle, mantled with ivy, still present a venerable appearance.

The inhabitants are celebrated for their romantic loyalty. After the Revolution, they presented an address to the king, begging his acceptance of 4*s*. in the pound land-tax, assuring him, that if the service required it, they would cheerfully add the other sixteen. The Dart here becomes a good river, and its banks, in many places, are highly picturesque.

BRADLEY.

This house, which retains its ancient gothic grandeur, unmixed with modern architecture, lies in a valley of the same name. The situation is picturesque, and well assimilates with the building. It is the property of Thomas Lane, esq.

TORR ABBEY

Was built by William Lord Brewer, in the reign of King John. Some of its original arches and windows remain; but the mansion which occupies its site is comparatively modern. The Roman Catholic chapel attached to the house is ornamented with a superb altar, and two capital paintings. The mansion consists of a centre and two wings, fronting the most captivating part of Torbay, and is surrounded by tall avenues of luxuriant growth.

KENT'S HOLE.

About half a mile beyond Torwood, a fine old seat of sir Lawrence Palk, in a coppice, lies the celebrated cavern called Kent's Hole, the opening of which is of moderate dimensions, and almost hid in bushes. Within, however, it contains chasms and intricate windings, which no stranger should attempt to explore without a guide. Petrifactions and incrustations adorn the roof and sides; but the whole is dark and dreary, and, in some places, scarcely high enough to allow a person to stand erect.

Not long since, some naval officers, rashly venturing into this horrid cavern without a guide, their lights became extinguished; and, had not one of them found his way out, and returned with assistance to his companions, it is probable they might have been buried alive in this cimmerian retreat.

COMPTON CASTLE.

This place, which is very ancient, and is now the property of James Templer, esq. contends with Haye's Farm, near Exmouth, for being the birthplace of sir Walter Raleigh. It is considerably modernized, but still retains much of its gothic grandeur. The ivy, twining round, and supporting the dilapidated walls of the once proud apartments, gives a sombre tinge to the spot, which even the view of the inhabited part is incapable of dissipating.

BERRY CASTLE.

Of this once proud fortress, which, from its advantageous situation, must have been nearly impregnable before the invention of artillery, little now remains, except its gateway and tower. It was long the baronial castle of the De Pomeroys, who had no less than fifty-eight lordships bestowed on them by the Conqueror. It occupies the whole of a projecting eminence, accessible only towards the south: and here it was defended strongly.

About the year 1556, the castle and its precincts became the property of the Seymours, one of whom began a magnificent edifice within the walls, which, however, was never completed. Berry-castle is a scene of unrivalled beauty; and the antiquary and the painter will here be gratified to the full, and unite in their admiration, though on different principles.

TORBAY.

Many other charming situations and picturesque landscapes will be visited by every person of taste, and particularly Torbay will not be omitted, which, besides its natural beauties, has oftentimes to boast of sheltering the channel fleet, the glory and defence of the British empire. Here, in a retiring cove, stands Torquay, a little fishing village, which has recently become a bathing-place.

The whole curve of Torbay is computed at twelve miles, between two capes, called Hope's Nose and Berry Head. Torquay is about two miles distant from the former, and is sheltered from the waves by a ridge of rocks. The air of this place is sharp; but, in romantic beauty and picturesque scenery, it cannot be surpassed; and those who can dispense with assembly-rooms and fashionable dissipations, may pass a few weeks in the summer at this sequestered spot, with satisfaction and improvement in health. At Brixham, on the western side of the bay, William Prince of Orange landed, November 5th, 1688. Here is a remarkable well, which ebbs and flows several times a day.

TENBY, in SOUTH WALES.

This rapidly improving bathing-place, which lies in the county of Pembroke, at the distance of 250 miles from London, and 60 from Swansea, is remarkable for the picturesque beauty of its situation, the romantic wildness of its rocks, and the excellent condition of its extensive sands.

GENERAL DESCRIPTION.

Tenby is a small, but a pleasant and populous, town, seated on the western edge of the fine bay of Carmarthen, and has a good harbour, capable of sheltering vessels from two to three hundred tons burthen. The houses are built of stone, and are covered with a blue slate, which gives the place a singular appearance in the approach to it by the Carmarthen road. At the distance of about half a mile from the entrance, the town breaks suddenly on the sight, seated on a bold and lofty peninsula, and nearly surrounded by the sea, while the distant coasts of Glamorgan, Devon, and Somerset, with the islands of Lundy and Caldy, give a beautiful effect to the picture. On descending into the town, the bay, castles, and pier, present themselves in an agreeable manner to the eye; and on the land-side, the ancient walls, flanked with towers, bear testimony to the antiquity and strength of the place. The extent of the wall, on the land-side, which encloses only a part of the town, is five hundred and twelve yards, and the height about twenty-one feet: this is furnished with embrasures, and flanked by two square and half-moon towers. The southernmost wall, seated on a rock, rises seventy-seven feet above the level of the sea at high water: and through one of the semi-circular towers, which is now fitted up as a depôt for government stores, is an entrance into the town,

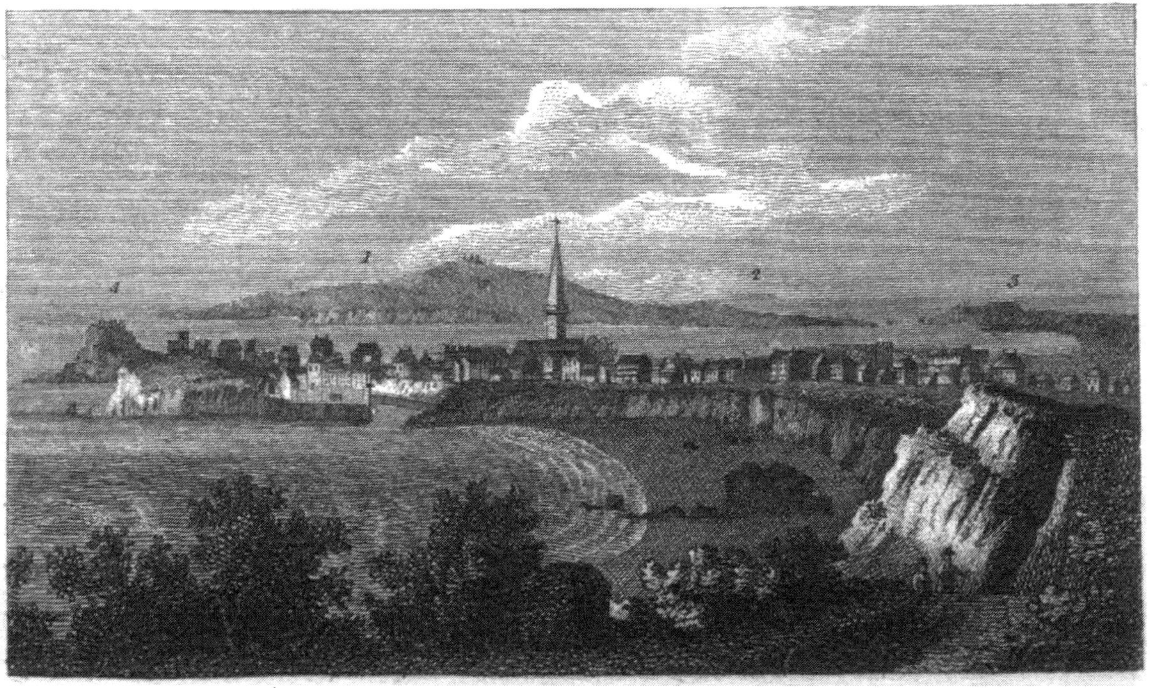

1 _ Isle of Caldy.
2 _ ___ _ Lundy.

Tenby.

3 _ Giltar . . . .
4 _ St. Catherine's & Castle.

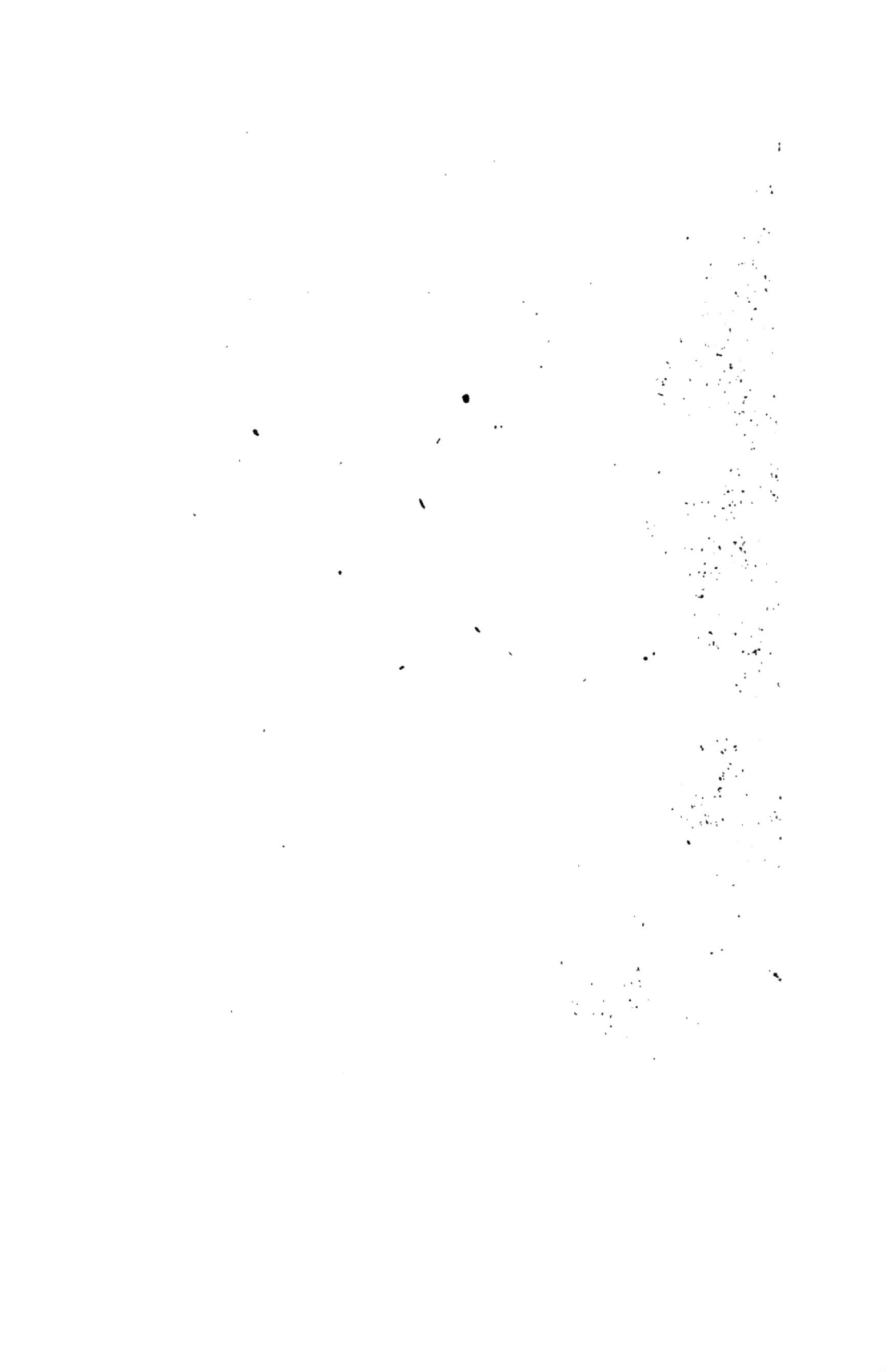

by a passage called the South-gate, formerly defended by an iron portcullis. The North-gate having fallen into decay, has been removed, so that the old town, as it is called, and the Norton or North-town, form one continued street, about three quarters of a mile in length. Besides these gateways, there are two more on the sea-side, one leading to the Pier, and the other to the South-sand. This sand, which is nearly three miles long, affords either an agreeable walk or ride, being perfectly firm, spacious, smooth, and easy. Here horse-races are occasionally held. The bold projecting rocks, the romantic islet of St. Catherine, which may be approached at low water, and the various prospects to be seen from the promontory, which extends nearly half a mile into the sea, all contribute to render this a favourite spot to every admirer of the sublimities of nature.* On a rock over these sands is a battery of eight long eighteen pounders, commanding their whole extent to the westward, and protecting the entrance through the sounds between the isle of St. Margaret and the main. Another battery of two guns, of the same calibre, is placed on the noble peninsular knowle called Castle-hill, which covers the Pier, and bounds the eastern extremity of these sands; this battery is calculated either to defend the shipping in the road, or to flank the fire with the other battery.

To the north, in the front of the town, is another excellent beach of sand, where the bathing-machines are kept. The gentle and almost imperceptible descent of this beach, and the great purity of the water, which flows immediately from the western ocean, unpolluted by the discharge of any river or stream, together with the salubrity of the air, free from fogs, marshy vapours, or any offensive streams, have contributed to render Tenby a fashionable place of re-

* There is another approach to the promontory of Giltar, by a pleasant walk along the Pembroke road, through the village of Pynally.

sort in the summer months, to those who have the combined objects of pleasure and health in view.

High above these sands, and adjoining Shaw's hotel, the company promenade, as this spot commands the prospect of a spacious expanse of water, on which numerous sails are continually passing and repassing.

THE CHURCH.

Tenby is a vicarage of moderate value, in the patronage of the Prince of Wales. The church, which is dedicated to the Virgin Mary, is a spacious structure, being 146 feet in length, and 83 in breadth.—The tower contains a set of six excellent bells, and on the east side is fixed the public clock. On the tower, is a lofty and elegant spire of Bath-stone, which from its elevated situation and colour, being painted white for its preservation, may be seen at the distance of several leagues: this is particularly mentioned, in order to rectify an error introduced into a late publication, which states that this spire is made of wood.

The roof of the church is supported by arcades, having fluted pillars: there are three aisles and a chancel, in which are some monuments, but none of them remarkable. The altar-piece is neat, and the steps to the communion-table, which are of Purbeck-stone, are rather elegant. Contiguous to the west door is an ancient edifice, now a school-room, which has over one of its windows the date, cut in stone, of 1496, and over the west door are the arms of the house of Lancaster.

CORPORATION, &C.

Tenby is governed by a mayor and two other magistrates, and an unlimited number of aldermen and burgesses, who in conjunction with the boroughs of Pembroke and Wiston, return one member to parliament. The charter, first granted by King John, has been considerably extended by succeeding monarchs, particularly Queen Elizabeth and Charles the First, whereby the inhabitants enjoy some peculiar privileges; such as being freed from the jurisdiction of the sheriff of the county, and from being impannelled on juries out of the town. Quarterly courts of session are held here, and the power vested in the three magistrates, who compose the same, is considerable. The authority of coroner in all cases of public inquest, within the town and its precincts, is wholly in the mayor.

TRADE.

The trade of Tenby consists of coal and culm, and the oyster and trawle-fisheries. The first is carried on by vessels from thirty to a hundred and fifty tons burthen, who convey coals and culm to various places in the Bristol, Irish, and British channels, and even to London. They take in their cargoes at Sandersfoot, three miles from Tenby, and at a few other places. The quantity usually exported amounts to about forty-five thousand tons in a year, there having cleared out at Tenby Custom-house 539 vessels in the year 1803.

As to the oyster-fishery, which has been long established, being mentioned as standing in high repute in the reign of Elizabeth, it now yields a supply of from thirty to forty thousand in a day, vast quantities of them being shipped for Liverpool and Bristol, and others are pickled and sent in jars to London and other places. The trawle-fishery, which, from April to October, is carried on by about fifteen smacks of thirty tons each, afford an abundant supply, not only to this and the adjacent places, but also to the Bristol and Bath markets.

ACCOMMODATIONS AND AMUSEMENTS.

Shaw's long-established hotel is well situated, a little within the entrance of the town, and affords excellent entertainment. Jenkins's hotel, recently fitted up with every accommodation, for the reception of genteel families, is in the centre of the town, and commands a charming prospect of the bay, pier, castle, and the north sands. Next to it is the Lyon Inn, standing on the most elevated part of the town, and enjoying every advantage which so airy a situation, and an extensive sea-prospect, can afford.—Here the assemblies are held weekly, on Wednesday, and are generally full and fashionably attended.—The Ball Inn, though not so happily situated, has many conveniences to recommend it. Good private lodgings, well supplied, and accompanied by that peculiar hospitality which distinguishes the principality of Wales, may be met with in every part of the town: and entire houses furnished may be had at five or six guineas a week, and private lodgings at half those sums.

Tenby has been greatly improved in its internal state, since it became a place of public resort.—The streets, which were formerly ill-paved, narrow, and exceedingly dirty, are now rendered smooth, and kept clean, and in several parts they have been idened.

In addition to the weekly assemblies, are a theatre, bowling-green, billiard-table, and a public card assembly-room. These, with frequent routes given by private parties, with aquatic excursions, form the round of fashionable amusement at this place.

THE LIBRARY.

Mr. Griffiths has an excellent Circulating Library here, well supplied with new publications, and his terms are exceedingly moderate. Here also the London papers are received for the accommodation of subscribers.

RIDES, &c.

The road to Pembroke, commonly called the Ridgeway, furnishes a most delightful ride of ten miles in length. On one side lies the rich vale of St. Florence, and, on the other side, the eye is presented with the bold rocky shore, and a fine view of the sea. Pembroke itself is a place which excites no particular interest, except from its vicinity to Milford Haven; the finest harbour in the world. Hitherto this neighbourhood has not been sufficiently frequented by travellers, in quest of pleasure, to render it worth the while of any person upon the Haven to supply parties with pleasure-boats.—Some fine views of this noble harbour may, however, be obtained from various eminences, in the vicinity of Pembroke.

STACKPOOLE COURT, &c. &c.

Stackpoole Court, the seat of Lord Cawdor, three miles to the south of Pembroke, is another object for a morning's ride. The house and grounds are equal to any thing of the kind in Pembrokeshire. Other seats deserving of notice are Ivy Tower, belonging to Mr. Williams; Kilgotty; the mansion of Lord Milford; Lawrenny Hall, a handsome house, the property of Hugh Barlow, esq. commanding a fine prospect of Milford Haven; and Ambroth House, the seat of James Ackland, esq.; Manor-beer Castle, about five miles, and Carew Castle, about seven miles from Tenby towards Pembroke, exhibit magnificent ruins; and the situation of the village, castle, and bay, of Manor-beer, is highly romantic.

North-east from Tenby, the road to Sander's-foot Bay, about four miles over the hills, furnishes a pleasant and highly picturesque ride. Here is a house of entertainment, from which, at low water, may be viewed one of the busiest scenes in this part of the world, in the loading of various vessels with coals; an employment in which several hundred persons are actively engaged. Lord Milford is the principal owner of these coal-pits. The coals are such as are preferred for lime-kilns and malt-houses.

Among the various scenery, the prospect from the hill on the road, where Tenby first bursts upon the sight, deserves attention. In fine weather, the opposite coast of Devonshire, and the island of Lundy, may be clearly described.

ISLES OF CALDY AND ST. MARGARET.

One of the most picturesque and interesting objects, in its relation to Tenby, is the island of Caldy, situated about three miles from the shore. This island furnishes pleasant aquatic excursions to persons fond of sailing, and convenient boats may, at all times, be hired for the purpose, at an expence of from 10*s.* to 15*s.*

Caldy is, at present, the property of Mr. Kynaston, who has a convenient dwelling there, with cottages for labourers. It is about three miles long, and one and a half broad, and is chiefly remarkable for its breed of rabbits. To persons used to cultivated landscapes, the wildness of the cliffs, and of the surrounding scenery, will not fail to afford a most agreeable novelty. Separated from Caldy, by an abrupt chasm, obviously occasioned by some convulsion of nature, is the small rocky island called the Margarets, the sole inhabitants of which are swarms of rabbits. These two islands add greatly to the picturesque effect of all the adjoining scenery.

Good saddle-horses may be hired on easy terms, at several places in the town; but carriages, or post-chaises, cannot be procured nearer than Narbeth, Tavernspite, or Pembroke. Persons who keep their own carriages usually travel to Tenby with post-horses. Good post-chaises may be met with either by the upper road of Monmouth and Brecknock; or by the lower road of Cardiff and Swansea. The only public conveyance from London is the Milford mail, from the Swan with Two Necks, which runs through, Narbeth (ten miles from Tenby) every day about two o'clock in the afternoon. There is also a coach through Gloucester and Brecknock, as far as Carmarthen, which runs three times a week, from the Bolt-in-tun, Fleet-street.

The post arrives with letters from London and other places about seven o'clock in the evening, in the sum-

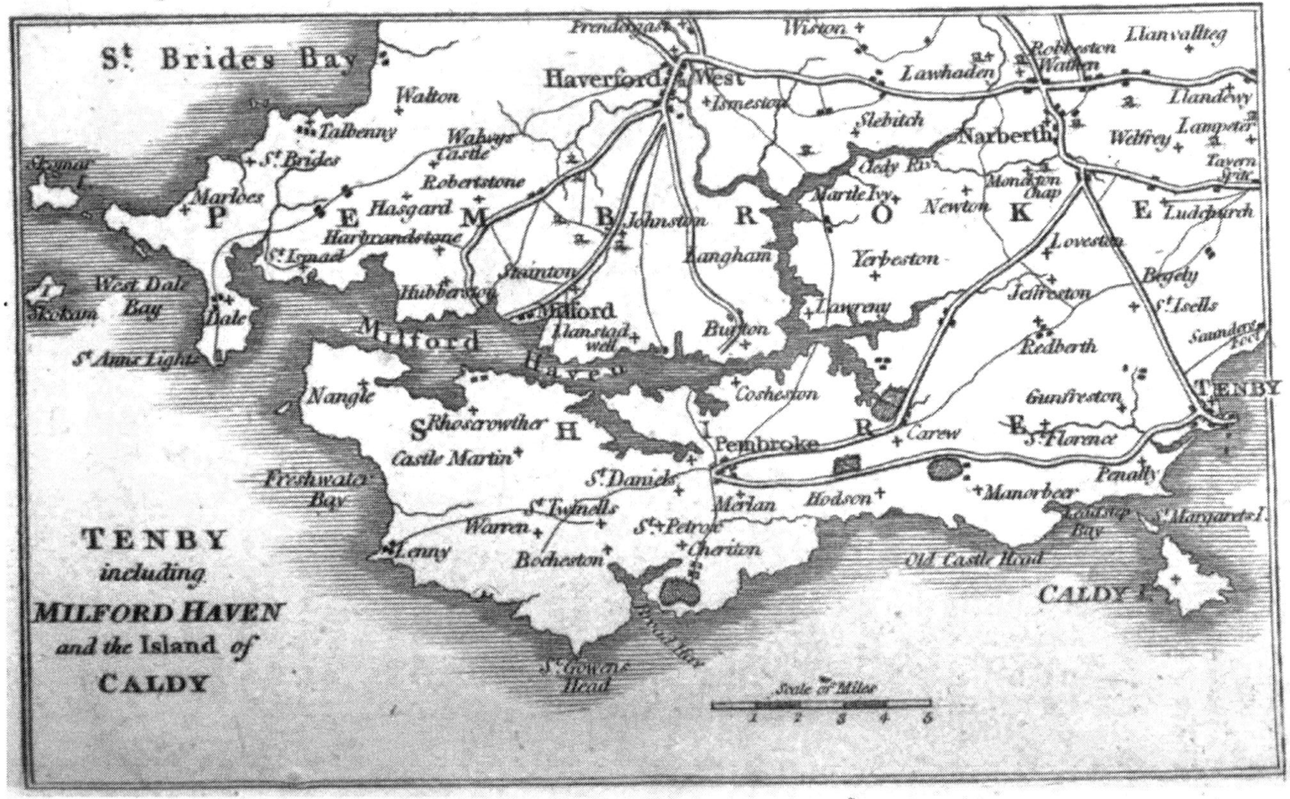

St. Brides Bay
Haverford West
Walton
Talbenny
St. Brides
Marloes
Robertstone
Hasgard
Johnston
Langham
Slebitch
Narberth
Lawhaden
Wiston
Llanvallteg
Llandewy
Welfrey
Lampeter
Newton
Yerbeston
Lawreny
Burton
Milford
Milford Haven
Nangle
Castle Martin
Pembroke
Cosheston
Carew
Redberth
Gunfreston
St. Florence
Manorbeer
Penally
Tenby
Caldy I.
Old Castle Head
Hodson
Merlan
St. Daniels
St. Twinells
Warren
Lenny
Bocheston
Cheriton
St. Petrox
Freshwater Bay
West Dale Bay
Dale
St. Anns Light
Skokum
Skomar I.
Ludchurch
St. Issells
Begely
Jeffreston
Loveston
St. Margarets I.
St. Gowens Head
Scale of Miles
1 2 3 4 5
P E M B R O K E
TENBY
including
MILFORD HAVEN
and the Island of
CALDY

mer months; but in the winter the arrival is uncertain, as it depends much on the state of the weather, the condition of the roads, and on the time of the mail's crossing the passage. The post sets out again the following morning to meet the mail-coach at Narbeth.

The Tenby season usually commences in May, and closes about the latter end of October. The company, of late years, has been numerous and fashionable; many persons, of the highest distinction, having taken houses for several successive seasons. In a word, Tenby may be considered as one of the most delightful summer retreats, and as a place which is every year increasing in publicity and convenience.

The following are the terms of bathing, exclusive of towels and attendants:—COLD BATH. Private, each person, 1*s.* 3*d.*; ditto, if more in a family, each 1*s.*; swimming bath, 9*d.*; shower-bath, 1*s.* 3*d.* WARM BATH.—Each person, 2*s.* 6*d.*; children, each, 2*s.* 6*d.*; vapour bath, 3*s.* The baths are ready at all hours of the day or night; the warm bath at three quarters of an hour's notice. The water is remarkably clear, and the bottom is excellent.

TUNBRIDGE WELLS.

Among mineral waters of the chalybeate kind, those of Tunbridge have long maintained distinguished pre-eminence; and the place owes no less to the virtues of its springs, than to the accommodations it offers to visitors, and to central situation, being only thirty-six miles distant from the metropolis.

SITUATION.

Tunbridge Wells lie in a sandy bottom, closely surrounded by steep hills, which contract the atmosphere, and diminish the elasticity of the air. The general aspect of the country is little inviting; and, but for its salutary springs, and its artificial allurements, few would be inclined to select it for their residence.

The general appellation of Tunbridge Wells is given to a few villages and dwellings within five or six miles from the town of Tunbridge, on the southern side of the county of Kent, on the borders of Sussex. They are situate in the three parishes of Tunbridge, Frant, and Speldhurst; and consist of four divisions, Mount Ephraim, Mount Pleasant, Mount Sion, and the Wells, properly so called.

THE WELLS:

THEIR QUALITIES AND VIRTUES.

That part, by way of distinction, called the Wells, is the centre of business and amusement; because here rise the springs, here the markets are held, and here the chapel, the assembly-rooms, and the public parades are exhibited.

The discovery of the medicinal waters at Tunbridge is generally ascribed to Dudley Lord North, a distinguished courtier in the reign of James I. This nobleman, having injured his constitution by fashion-

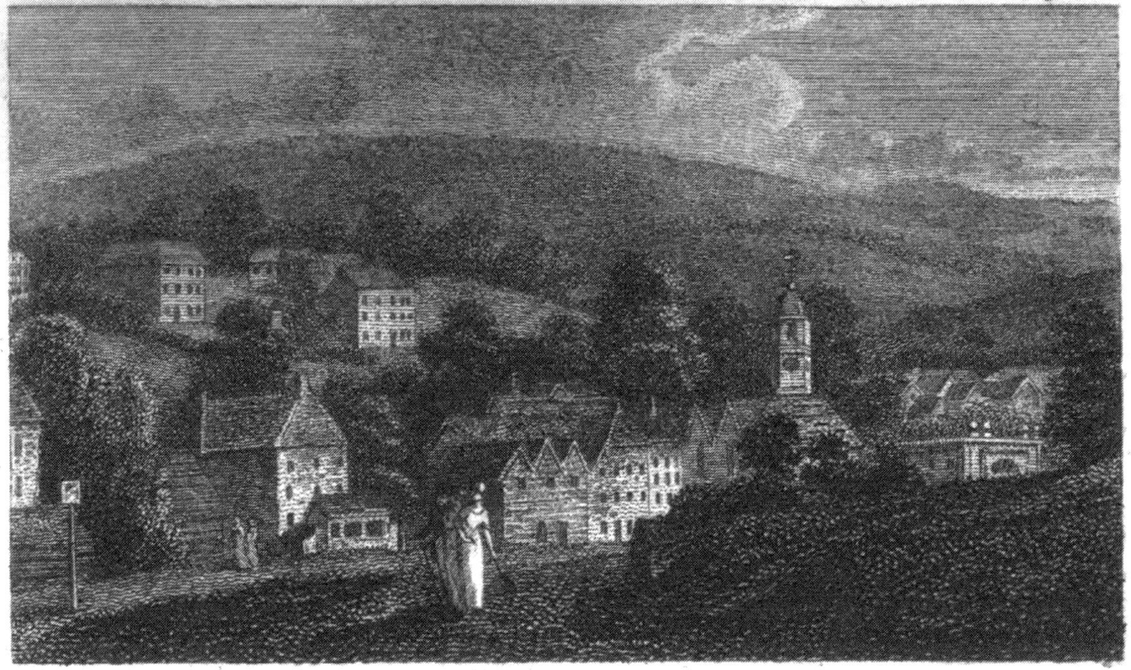

Tunbridge Wells.

able excesses, was advised, as a last resource, to retire into the country. Having fixed his residence at Edridge house, about two miles off, he remained there some time, with little improvement in his health. Determined to leave this sequestered spot, and to return to London, fortunately for him, his way lay through a wood, where he observed the water, that has since become so famous, with a mineral scum on its surface, and an earthy sediment at bottom. His genius suggested to him, that this might furnish the tonic his case required; and, on consulting his physicians, they advised a trial. In the space of three months after he commenced the use of the waters, his lordship's health was perfectly restored, and his debilitated frame so completely invigorated, that he lived to be eighty-five years of age.

It is proper, however, to add, that the authority on which this account rests is rendered somewhat doubtful, from the circumstance of its not being mentioned by lord North, in his work entitled The Forest of Varieties, though his lordship mentions Epsom Wells.

The reputation of the waters being established, invalids began to resort to them; and Lord Abergavenny, having an estate in the vicinity, exerted himself to provide proper accommodations for visitors. The springs were cleared out and secured; and, during the summer season, Tunbridge town, about six miles distant, and the nearest place where lodgings could be procured, was crowded.

By degrees, buildings arose in the immediate vicinity of the Wells, and other improvements were adopted to render them convenient, as well for the votaries of health, as for those of pleasure.

It would be tedious to enumerate the progressive steps that were taken to attract company to Tunbridge Wells, and to particularize the royal and noble personages who have patronized them Suffice it to say, that the place is now in the most flourishing state; that its customs are settled, its pleasures regulated, and every provision made that can render it conducive to the purposes for which it claims public regard.

Chalybeate springs are common in this district: but, as the properties of all are nearly the same, only the two first discovered are held in particular estimation. These are enclosed with a new triangular stone wall, containing a well-paved area, which is entered by a handsome gateway. Over the springs are placed basons, with perforations at the bottom, and an opening in the edge to discharge the overflowings.

The water at the fountain head is extremely clear and pellucid. It has little smell, but the taste is strongly impregnated with iron.

From the experiments of physicians it appears, that the component parts of this water are—steely particles, marine salts, an oily matter, an ochreous substance, a volatile vitriolic spirit, too subtle for analysis, and a simple fluid. In long continued rains, it acquires a milky appearance, but its effects are hereby little diminished.

Tunbridge water is excellently adapted to warm and invigorate the relaxed constitution, to restore the weakened fibres to their due tone and elasticity, to remove obstructions in the minuter vessels, and thereby to promote digestion, and an even flow of spirits. In a languid state of the circulation, and in nervous and female complaints in general, it seems to possess sovereign efficacy: but, in using it, the advice of a sensible physician should be taken. Of all mineral waters, iron is the most friendly to the human constitution, and this natural combination of it is, perhaps, preferable to any that art can produce; yet it may be laid down as a general maxim, "that what is calculated to do much good, may also do much harm;" and, therefore, judgment and care are necessary in the exhibition of all potent remedies.

A quarter of a pint will be enough for weak and delicate persons to begin with, which may be increas-

Page 436.

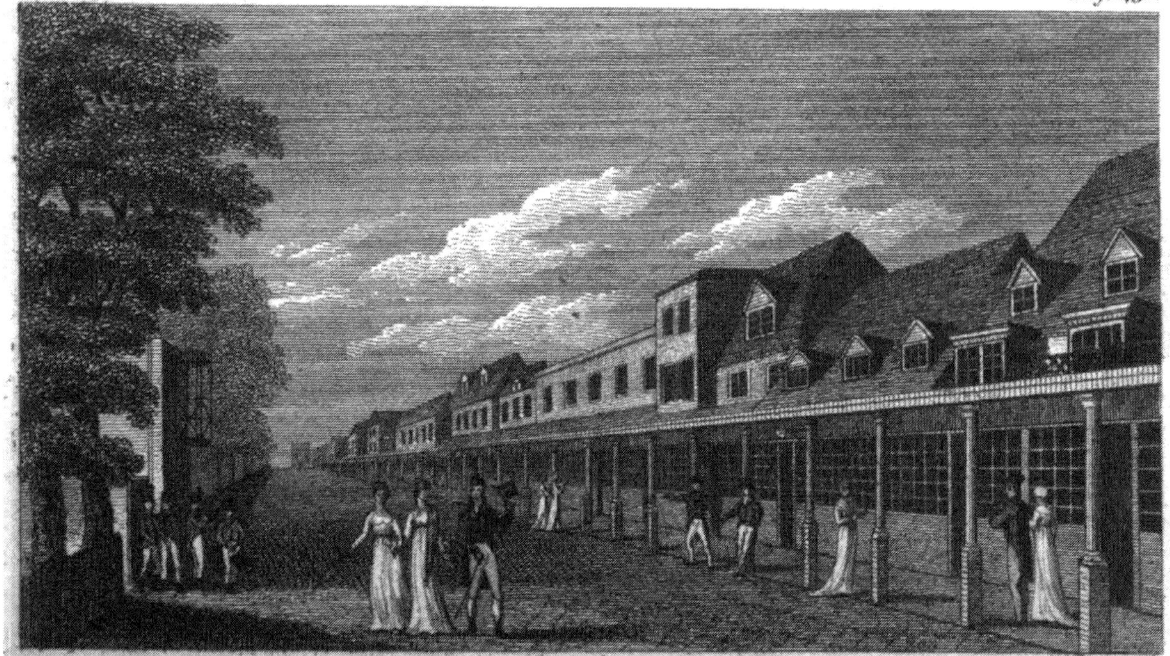

Parade, Tunbridge Wells.

ed to half a pint, or more; but this should be taken at equal draughts, at an interval of twenty minutes. Persons of stronger stamina may use double the quantity; yet it is always adviseable to begin with moderate doses, and towards the close of the course to diminish in the same proportion.

Temperance and exercise are indispensibly requisite to give the waters a chance of producing beneficial effects. Those persons however, who are labouring under chronic complaints, are subject to lassitude, and, by indulgence, confirm the evils which they came here to remove.

THE PARADES, PUBLIC-ROOMS, &c.

The parades, usually called the Upper and Lower Walk, run parallel to each other, and are much frequented. The former was once paved with pantiles, raised about four steps above the other; but, in 1793, it was paved by subscription with Purbeck-stone, at the expence of more than 700*l.* The Lower Walk is divided from it by a range of pallisadoes, and is chiefly used by servants and country people.

A portico, supported by wooden Tuscan pillars, runs the entire length of the principal walk, and affords an agreeable shelter from the sun and rain. A row of elms of luxuriant growth, also contributes to the amenity of the place; and, under the shade, the company meet, sit, or walk, during the hours of general resort.

One set of the Public Rooms stands on the right, and also the Libraries, Coffee-house, &c. with many neat little shops for the sale of jewellery, perfumery, and Tunbridge-ware. On the left of the street are other houses of entertainment, the lower set of Assembly-rooms, with a number of boarding and lodging-houses.

TAVERNS.

The three principal taverns are, the Sussex, the Kentish, and the New Inn and Tavern. The former, with the Lower Assembly-rooms, are occupied by the same person. Each furnishes good accommodation to travellers or visitors. The Angel Inn and Tavern, situate by the road side, on entering the place, is also extremely convenient for business.

MOUNT-SION HILL.

This delightful spot received its name from a landlord, of the name of Jordan, who building a house here, affixed to it the sign of Mount Sion. It is now composed chiefly of lodging-houses, so charmingly intermixed with trees and groves, and so well sheltered from the easterly winds, that they are generally well filled. We are told of a parish clerk, who had a house here, and who constantly gave out the Psalm that begins "Mount Sion is a pleasant place," till he had let it to his mind; but, after it was occupied, thought no more about his favourite, till he wanted another tenant.

MOUNT PLEASANT.

This spot justly deserves the name it has acquired. It contains, however, only three or four patrician houses with their accompaniments.

MOUNT EPHRAIM.

Mount Ephraim, situate about half a mile from the Wells, was once the most fashionable quarter, possessing its assembly-room, tavern, and bowling-green. These have disappeared, or been converted into private houses; but still it is a charming situation, and is much admired by those who are inclined to mingle retirement with public amusement.

BISHOP'S DOWN.

Though still more distant than Mount Ephraim, this place contains some good lodging-houses and private dwellings.

THEATRE.

Of the theatre, little can be said. It is small, but often well filled: and, if those who tread its stage are not of the first order of merit, they do not deserve to be classed in the lowest.

CHAPEL, CHARITY-SCHOOL, &c.

Towards the close of the seventeenth century, when Tunbridge Wells began to draw company from various quarters, a place of public worship was found necessary, and a liberal subscription was raised for erecting a chapel, in which divine service is performed every day during the season, and thrice a week in winter. The clergyman, however, has no other endowment, except the voluntary subscription of the company during summer, and of the fixed inhabitants during winter. This subscription is calculated to amount to near 300*l.* a year, a sum certainly not contemptible; but it is to be lamented that it does not arise from a more permanent and creditable source. It is mortifying to a man of education and religious principle, to be paid for his prayers, like a master of the ceremonies for his obsequious bows and attentions.

Adjoining the chapel, which is large and commodious, is a charity-school, for fifty or more boys and girls, who are instructed by the chapel clerk. This benevolent institution is chiefly supported by a contribution collected at the chapel doors.

Dissenters of various denominations have their meetings at Tunbridge Wells; and the Methodists, in particular, are numerous and active.

TRADE.

The trade carried on here is similar to that of the Spa, in Germany, and consists chiefly of toys, and useful domestic articles, in wood. Great quantities of these are sold to the company; and also in different parts of the kingdom. The elegance of these articles is universally admired. They are generally made of cherry-tree, plum-tree, yew, and sycamore.

ACCOMMODATIONS.

Tunbridge Wells furnishes excellent lodgings for persons of condition; but those which can be hired by the middling or lower classes of society are neither numerous nor very agreeable. Provisions, however, are reasonable; and the epicure will be delighted to find that his favourite wheat-ear may be had here in perfection.

A daily post is established between this place and London: the morning and evening newspapers likewise reach the Wells a few hours after publication; stage-coaches pass and repass to the metropolis every day; and, in addition to these extrinsic advantages, the resident inhabitants are reckoned civil and obliging, and not particularly addicted to exaction—a rare quality at an established watering-place.

AMUSEMENTS.

The celebrated Nash once presided over the amusements at Tunbridge Wells, and some of his institutions still remain in force.

On arrival, every person who intends to drink the waters, takes a glass, and pays what is called a "welcome penny" to the dippers. He then subscribes at the Libraries, which are well filled, also at the Coffee-house, and at the Assembly-rooms. The Band of Music, and the Clergyman, have likewise their separate books; and, after a person has put down his name at each place enumerated, he may consider himself as privileged to join in the amusements of the place.

The company generally assemble on the parade pretty early in the morning; and, after drinking the water, and spending an hour or two in walking, frequently assemble in parties to breakfast. After this repast, it is customary to attend morning service in the chapel, and to walk, ride, or read, according to the predominant disposition.

Prayers over, the music re-commences, and the walks become crouded with those who have an inclination to distant excursions, or select society. Dinner over, the band again ascends the orchestra, and the evening promenade commences, which is only interrupted by tea, the theatre, card-assemblies, or the public rooms.

The Master of the Ceremonies has two balls in the season, which are generally very brilliant and full.

Private balls too are frequently given by people of fashion in the height of the season; and on these occasions elegant suppers are generally superadded.

Here also are frequent concerts, attended by the most eminent performers in London. Sometimes these concerts form a part of the morning amusement, under the name of concert breakfasts, and then the price of tickets, which are commonly 5s. seldom exceed 3s. 6d.

Another species of Tunbridge amusement consists in parties to the High Rocks,* and other romantic scenes, with which the whole neighbourhood abounds. At these places there frequently are public breakfasts, dinners, and tea-drinkings, attended with music and dancing.

Excursions to the noblemen's and gentlemen's seats, the founderies, and many remarkable places in the adjacent country, some of which will be particularized, furnish another pleasureable employment of time at Tunbridge Wells. There are, indeed, several capital houses in the vicinity, which, through

* These rocks are about a mile and a half southward from the Wells, and consist of a great number of rude eminences adjacent, several of which are above seventy feet high, though their average may be taken at forty. Situate among woods, by the side of a gentle murmuring stream, they are at once romantic and sequestered, though by no means to be compared with the rich scenery of Matlock.

the polite hospitality of the worthy proprietors, are always open to the inspection of the curious; and there are many pleasant villages, and agreeable prospects, in the roads leading to them, that will not fail to please.

Above all, the more serious and reflecting part of the company will find the Circulating Libraries, and the Coffee-house, replete with the most rational amusement. The easy freedom, and cheerful gaiety, arising from the nature of a public place, extends its influence over them, and every species of party spirit is hushed into peace. Here divines and philosophers, whigs and tories, debate without anger, dispute with politeness, and judge with candour.

The bookseller's shop has, indeed, one advantage over the coffee-house, because there the ladies are admitted, to enhance the charms of society, and to diffuse a softer polish over the manners of the company.

The season at Tunbridge Wells, being now of much longer duration than formerly, some families come as early as March or April, and many continue here till the latter end of November; particularly those who come merely for the benefit of health, the water being reckoned equally beneficial in cold weather, provided it be dry; and the air, though sharp, as pure and healthy as in summer. It may be necessary to observe, that there are two resident apothecaries, in high repute, who are well acquainted with the qualities and effects of the waters; and a regular physician, or two, from London, constantly attends at the Wells, during the usual period of drinking this justly celebrated chalybeate, which combined with air, exercise, and regimen, has certainly done wonderful cures.

WALKS AND RIDES ROUND TUNBRIDGE WELLS.

SPELDHURST.

In this parish the chalybeate springs rise, though they obtain the name of Tunbridge Wells. The church here is a very ancient structure, and contains some curious monuments, particularly of the Waller family. In 1791, this sacred edifice was burnt down by lightning. Even the bells were melted by the intense heat.

Groombridge, in this parish, is a place of some note. It has passed through several noble families, and is now the seat of the Camfields.

GREAT BOUNDS.

This place receives its appellation from being the extreme boundary of the liberty of Tunbridge. It is about three miles from the Wells, and was lately the property and residence of lady Dowager Darnley. The house, which is a neat Gothic pile, commands very extensive views.

PENSHURST.

Five miles north-west of the Wells stands the little pleasant town of Penshurst, or the *Head of the Wood*, adjoining to which is Penshurst-place, a noble and ancient mansion, which has passed through many distinguished families, and is celebrated for having been the birth-place of the gallant and learned sir Philip Sidney, who fell at the battle of Zutphen, in the thirty-fifth year of his age; and also of that sturdy patriot, Algernon Sidney, who was beheaded in 1683.

Penshurst-place still remains in the Sidney family. It contains a noble collection of pictures. The gardens which are bounded by the Medway, are large and beautiful; and the park is of great extent, and charmingly diversified with hill and dale, woods and lawns.

Here mighty Dudley* once would rove,
To plan his triumphs in the grove;

* Earl of Leicester.

Here looser Waller, ever gay,
With Sacharissa in dalliance lay;
And Philips sidelong yonder spring,
His lavish carols wont to sing.

PENSHURST, a POEM.

In Penshurst church are several antique monuments. The Sidneys have been buried here for upwards of 200 years.

HEVER.

This place, which lies about seven or eight miles from the Wells, on the river Eden, is chiefly remarkable for its ancient castle, of which considerable ruins still remain. It was built in the time of Edward III. by William de Hever, and afterwards fell into the hands of the Bullens. On the execution of Queen Anne Bullen, and her brother, Lord Rochford, it became forfeited to the crown. It is now the property of sir Timothy Waldo, knt.

TUNBRIDGE.

This town, from which the Wells receive their name, lies about six miles distant from them. It was once so considerable as to send burgesses to parliament. It lies on the river Medway, and may be regarded as a flourishing town, containing many good houses and respectable inhabitants. The church is a handsome modern structure.

Tunbridge is famous for its grammar-school, founded by sir Andrew Judd, lord-mayor of London, in 1551.

Here stood a large castle, which is still magnificent in its ruins. It was the scene of many memorable events, during a long succession of ages, and its mouldering remains now furnish a topic on which the philosopher may moralize.

SOMERHILL.

About four miles from the Wells stands Somerhill, a large old mansion, on an elevated site, commanding a fine view of the country. It originally belonged to the earls of Hereford and Gloucester; Queen Elizabeth gave it to sir Francis Walsingham, whose daughter Frances carried it successively to her three husbands, sir Philip Sidney, the unfortunate earl of Essex, and the earl of Clanrickard.

The heir, at length, was Margaret Viscountess Purbeck, a woman of a most generous disposition. The house and estate now belong to the Woodgates.

This is a favourite ride from the Wells. In count Gramont's Memoirs are some entertaining anecdotes of the noble inhabitants of this place, at the time he wrote.

BAYHALL.

This neat and convenient mansion lies about three miles east of Tunbridge Wells. It was formerly the property of the Colepepers. After passing through various hands it came to the Amherst family. The house is pleasantly situated, in the midst of fine meadows, gardens, and fish-ponds.

FRANT.

Frant lies about two miles from the Wells. The church stands on a high hill. Here are several neat and modern-built houses, forming collectively a handsome village.

BAYHAM ABBEY.

About six miles from the Wells stands Bayham Abbey. It originally belonged to the Premonstratensians, or White Canons, so called from their dress.

The ruins of this venerable pile stand on an extensive level, and its romantic beauties attract the admiration of every spectator. Every where it displays massy richness of Gothic architecture, the preservation of which is indebted to the repairs it has received from the proprietors.

Seats are interspersed among the trees, where the visitor may contemplate at his ease, the changes that time has wrought: a branch of the Medway mur-

murs at the foot of the Abbey, and gives a finish to the pensive scenery.

The whole domain belongs to the Camden family; and the Gothic house, which has been built here, harmonizes with the rest of the scene.

COURT LODGE.

Near Lamberhurst, where a grand iron furnace has been long established, stands Court Lodge, a seat of the Morlands, once the venerable residence of Edward III. It has been much improved by its last possessor, and is generally visited by the company from the Wells.

EDRIDGE PARK.

This belongs to the Earl of Abergavenny, and lies within a short distance of the Wells, in the neighbourhood of Frant. It used to be open to respectable company, who were indulged with the liberty of riding in the park, which certainly possesses many natural beauties.

Within the circle of a morning's ride, many other places deserving notice might be indicated, and those who spend a summer at Tunbridge Wells will, doubtless, be inclined to visit them all.

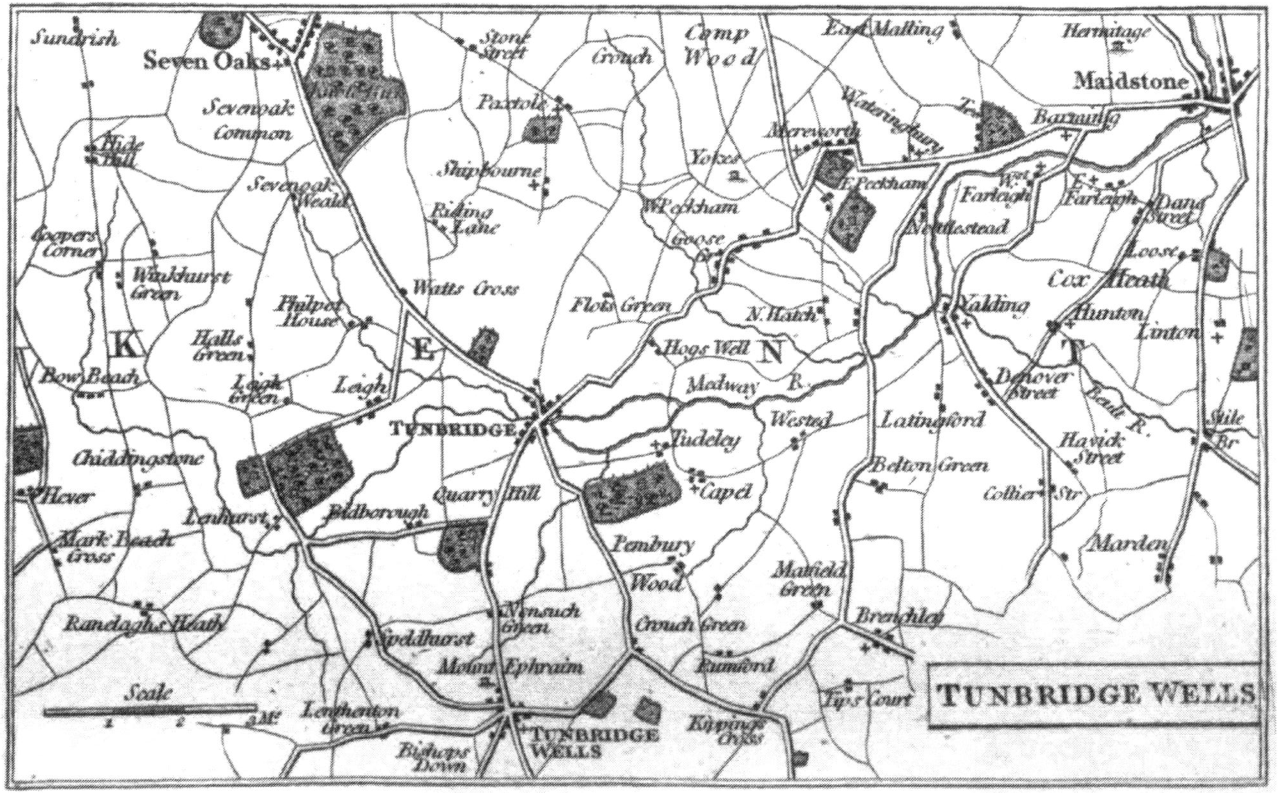
TUNBRIDGE WELLS
Sundrish
Seven Oaks
Sevenoak Common
Sevenoak Weald
Coopers Corner
Winkhurst Green
Philpot House
Halls Green
Bow Beach
Leigh
Chiddingstone
Hever
Mark Beach Cross
Ranelagh Heath
Lenhurst
Bidborough
Speldhurst
Mount Ephraim
Lentherton Green
Bishops Down
TUNBRIDGE WELLS
Stone Street
Paxtole
Shipbourne
Riding Lane
Watts Cross
TUNBRIDGE
Quarry Hill
Nonsuch Green
Pembury
Wood
Crouch Green
Rumford
Kippings Cross
Camp Wood
Crouch
Yokes
W. Peckham
Goose Green
Flols Green
Hogs Well
N. Hatch
Medway R.
Tudeley
Capel
Wested
Matfield Green
Brenchley
Tips Court
East Malling
Mereworth
Wateringbury
E. Peckham
Nettlestead
Yalding
Latingford
Belton Green
Hermitage
Maidstone
Barming
Wt. Farleigh
E. Farleigh
Dane Street
Loose
Cox Heath
Hunton
Linton
Denover Street
Beale R.
Havick Street
Collier Str
Marden
Stile Br
K
E
N
T
Scale
1
2
3 Ms

Pl. 41. P. 377

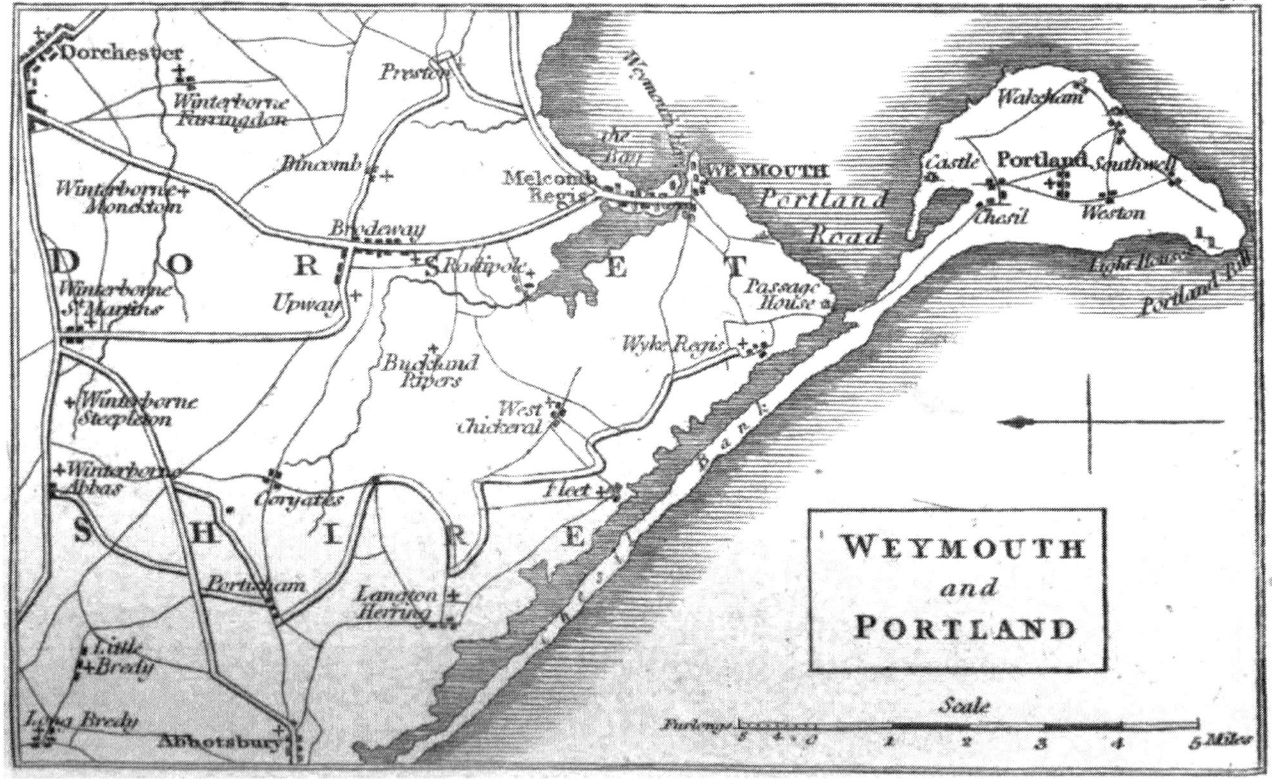
WEYMOUTH and PORTLAND
Dorchester
Winterborne Farringdon
Preston
Bincomb
Winterborne Monckton
Brodeway
Upway
Winterborne St. Martins
Radipole
Melcomb Regis
the Bay
WEYMOUTH
Portland Road
Passage House
Wyke Regis
Buckland Rivers
West Chickeral
Winterborne Steepleton
Winterborne Abbas
Coryates
Fleet
Portisham
Langton Herring
Little Brady
Long Bredy
Abbotsbury
Chesil Bank
D O R S E T
S H I R E
Castle
Portland
Southwell
Wakeham
Chesil
Weston
Light House
Portland Bill
Scale
Furlongs
5 Miles

WEYMOUTH.

Since their majesties, and other branches of the royal family, first visited Weymouth in 1749,* and have honoured it with an annual residence of some weeks, during the season, it has become one of the most fashionable of all the sea-bathing places.

SITUATION, POLITICAL HISTORY, RISE AND PROGRESS.

Weymouth, in Dorsetshire, distant about 128 miles from London, stands on the south-side of the river Wye, which separates it from the town of Melcombe Regis, on one of the finest bays in the world. It is a place of considerable antiquity, and has long been a borough town, as well as its neighbour, Melcombe Regis. As one borough, they now return four members to serve in parliament, a privilege allowed to no other place in the kingdom, except London. The representatives are elected by the freeholders of Weymouth and Melcombe, whether inhabitants or otherwise, and the successful candidates are returned in one indenture. The mayor is the returning officer. A good police is kept up here by the magistrates, who are ready to adopt every plan that can add to the improvement of the place.

Formerly Weymouth carried on a considerable trade, and was the principal port in the county, but it is now rivalled by Poole, and depends more on the company resorting to it, than on any commercial pursuits. Being sheltered by the sur-

* The late duke of Gloucester having passed the winter of 1780, at Weymouth, found his health so much improved, that he erected Gloucester Lodge, in the front of the bay, which having been since enlarged and improved, is the royal residence, during the bathing season.

rounding hills, possessing a pure salubrious air, a fine beach of sand, and a calm bay, forming a semicircle of more than two miles, it is extremely well adapted for the purpose of health and pleasure, and as a bathing-place it is almost unparallelled.

Till within the last twenty or thirty years, it was small and meanly built, but by rapid enlargements, and many elegant buildings, it is now become a very respectable place, with a population of 3600 souls. The most fashionable residences are Gloucester-row, Chesterfield-place, York-buildings, Charlotte-row, Augusta-place, St. Albans'-row, Clarence-buildings, and Belle Vue. These being in the vicinity of the rooms, the libraries, and the theatre, and commanding extensive views, both by sea and land, are held in general estimation by strangers as well as natives.

The celebrated Ralph Allen, esq. of Bath, recommended Weymouth as a bathing-place, about the year 1760, and the first machine seen on the beach was constructed for his use.

MARKETS, &c.

The market days here are Tuesdays and Fridays, when plenty of butcher's meat, poultry, and fish, may be purchased on reasonable terms. The small Portland mutton is met with in perfection; and the most delicate kinds of fish may be procured any day.

BATHING-MACHINES AND BATHS.

The place where the company bathe is the beautiful bay which lies in the front of the town, close to some of the most fashionable lodgings and places of public resort. Being protected from all winds, the sea here is remarkably tranquil; and hence, at all times of the day, immersion in the briny flood is safe and delightful. The sands are as smooth as a carpet, and solid to the tread, while the bathing-machines, upwards of thirty in number, are in constant requisition from six in the morning till noon. They are drawn into the sea by a horse, to the necessary depth, and are attended by proper guides on the usual terms, and in some cases under.

A commodious hot salt-water bath, on a large scale, is erected in a central part of the town, and deserves encouragement, not only on account of its utility in many cases of human infirmity, but from the manner in which it is fitted up and conducted. The price of a single bath is 3*s.* 6*d* if before six in the evening, and 4*s.* if after. A sedan-chair is kept in constant attendance.

There are, likewise, private cold baths, which many timid or infirm persons prefer to falling at once into the arms of Neptune. A superb bath of this description was erected as a speculation, for the use of his Majesty, but it was used only once, and the reason assigned was, that the water contained less of the marine salt than that on the beach.

THEATRE.

The business of the Weymouth stage is well conducted by Mr. Hughes. The house is elegantly fitted up, and the performers are frequently of the first order of merit. The best comedians from the London and Bath theatres, frequently exhibit their talents here, particularly during the residence of the royal family. The boxes are sufficiently large to accommodate 400 spectators.

PUBLIC ROOMS.

The public rooms and hotel, kept by Mr Stacie, stand in the centre of Gloucester-row.—The assembly-room is lofty, light, and spacious, and very handsomely decorated, as well as delightfully situated. The master of the ceremonies is Mr. Rodber, who has established the following regulations, by the common consent of his patrons.

I. That gentlemen are not to appear in the rooms, either on Tuesday or Friday evenings, in boots; nor ladies in riding-habits.

II. That the ball shall begin as soon as possible after seven o'clock, and finish precisely at eleven.

III. That ladies and gentlemen who dance down a country dance, shall not quit their place till the dance is finished, unless they do not mean to dance any more that night.

IV. That no lady or gentleman can be permitted to dance in coloured gloves.

V. That after a lady has called a dance, and danced it down, her place in the next dance is at the bottom.

VI. That no tea-table be carried into the card-room.

VII. That gentlemen will be pleased to leave their swords at the door.

VIII. That no dogs be admitted.

T. RODBER, M. C.

The terms of subscription are:

	£.	s.	d.
To the rooms, for the assemblies, during three seasons, three tickets, transferable	2	2	0
A single ticket, transferable	1	1	0
A gentleman for walking the rooms	0	10	6
A lady, ditto	0	5	0

LIBRARIES.

The principal library is near the centre of the Esplanade, and contains a good collection of books, with a commodious room for reading the newspapers. The card-room over the library is large, and elegantly furnished.

At another library on the Esplanade, besides a large stock of books, musical instruments may be hired, and all the fashionable articles of perfumery, &c. are kept on constant sale.

In a word, the lovers of reading will have no reason to complain that they cannot enjoy their favourite amusement at Weymouth; and even those who are satisfied with the exterior of books, will be gratified with a lounge in the elegant apartments where they are kept.

THE CHURCH.

Though Weymouth is a place of antiquity, it contains no buildings of a remote period, worthy the attention of the curious. The church, dedicated to St. Mary, consists of three aisles, but it is a low building. The altar-piece, however, the masterly production of sir James Thornhill, the celebrated painter of the cupola of St. Paul's, and of the Halls of Greenwich Hospital, and Blenheim, is universally admired. A good organ was erected here in 1797, by voluntary subscription. The place of organist was properly bestowed on an ingenious and amiable young lady, a native of the town.

LODGING AND BOARDING-HOUSES.

The principal lodging-houses are in Gloucester-buildings, Chesterfield-place, York-buildings, Charlotte-row, Augusta-place, East-street, the Esplanade, Clarence-place, Belle Vue; on the Quay, or South-parade, St. Edmund's-street, New-street, Maiden-street, St. Mary's-street, St. Thomas's-street.

There are also several commodious and well-furnished lodging-houses on both sides of the harbour, and in the interior of the town; but these are seldom taken till the apartments fronting the sands are all engaged.

The price, though in some measure regulated by the number of rooms, is high. Half price, however, is taken from the 21st of October to the 15th of June; and single gentlemen may generally be accommodated in pleasant situations, at all seasons, on moderate terms.

For the reception of those who dislike inns, or expensive establishments of their own at private houses, boarding-houses have been established, where ladies and gentlemen may be accommodated during the season, on reasonable terms, exclusive of tea, sugar, and wine. The most frequented boarding-houses are Scriven's, on the Esplanade, and Dymond's, behind the church.

INNS AND TAVERNS.

Since Weymouth has become a place of fashionable resort, its houses of entertainment have increased in proportion, and their elegance has been adapted to the rank of the company. The Hotel in Gloucester-row, the Hotel and Navy Tavern, the King's Head Inn, the Crown Inn, the Golden Lion, and the Bear Inn, are all good houses.

POST-OFFICE, PACKETS, &c.

The post-office, situate in St. Thomas's-street, is kept by Mrs. Delamotte. The post sets out daily for London at eleven o'clock in the morning, except Saturdays, and arrives every day at Weymouth by three in the afternoon, except Mondays. There are also bye-posts to the west of England, &c.

Two packets are stationed here for the islands of Guernsey and Jersey, one of which sails every Saturday with the mail and passengers, and returns about Wednesday or Thursday.

To London there are several coaches daily; and every other day, during the season, there is one to Bath and Bristol.

In time of peace, a trip to the Continent, to the islands of Guernsey, Jersey, and Alderney, is not unfrequent, and here company may be accommodated with excellent yachts and experienced navigators.

NOTTINGTON MINERAL SPRING.

At the distance of twelve furlongs from the turnpike, on the left of the Dorchester road, lies the small hamlet of Nottington, famous for its medicinal spring, which has been found extremely serviceable in cutaneous and scorbutic disorders. It has a strong sulphureous smell, though perfectly limpid, and acts chiefly on the urinary passages. It appears from analysis to contain hepatic, phlogisticated, and fixed air, the digestive salt of Sylvius, vegetable alkali, magnesia, &c. and strongly resembles the Moffatt water in Scotland. Combined with sea-bathing, under the direction of a judicious physician, it promises to be extremely efficacious in many cases of human infirmity.

PUBLIC WALKS.

As the Steyne is the fashionable promenade at Brighton, so the Esplanade is at Weymouth. It is about half a mile long, and thirty feet broad, from whence the company may descend to the sands, and walk with as much comfort as on a carpet, while the invigorating sea-breezes are playing round them.

From the centre of the bridge, which connects Weymouth and Melcombe Regis, the views up and down the river are pleasing, and from thence along the Quay to the end of the New Pier, is an amusing saunter, replete with variety.

At the extremity of this pier, which commands an uninterrupted view of the Esplanade, the Sands, and the Bay, various pleasure vessels are stationed, which may be hired for aquatic excursions. From this spot too their majesties also embark, when they go on board one of the ships of war, which attends here during their stay; and, on such an occasion, every yacht and boat in the harbour is filled with persons eager to accompany them in their progress.

To the Look-out, on the Weymouth side of the water, is another agreeable walk, commanding a beautiful view of the West Bay, the Isle of Portland, &c. This is frequently resorted to, as well for the view it furnishes, as because it is but a small distance from any part of the town.

A little to the left of the Look-out is the Camera Obscura, for the amusement of *great* children; and in the vicinity are a battery of heavy cannon, and horse-barracks.

A small distance from thence are the ruins of Weymouth, or Sandsford Castle; from which, to the Ferry-house, when the tide is out, the walk over the sands is equally salubrious and pleasant.

To the lovers of picturesque scenery, a walk to the villages of Wyke and Chickerill, will afford high gratification. Fresh beauties open at every step; the land and sea views are equally delightful, and the spectator of taste is rivetted to the spot.

The roads towards Dorchester and Wareham have also their appropriate beauties. The little village of Radipole, where stands the ancient mother church of Melcombe Regis, is rural and inviting.

But after all, the country appears naked from a deficiency of trees, and the traveller, panting under the meridian sun, sighs in vain for shade.

AQUATIC EXCURSIONS.

Many persons pass up the creek through Weymouth bridge to Radipole, where they will find a decent house of entertainment. This little excursion, however, can be taken only at spring tides, as there is not sufficient water at other times.

To Portland by water, the distance is not more than three miles, which may frequently be accomplished in half an hour, when wind and tide are favourable.

Barn Door, or Durdle Rock, on the north shore, is a surprising rock projecting from the cliffs towards the south, in form of a quadrant, and forming a little bay with the shore. The back part of the rock is extremely rough and uneven; and the inside, which preserves the same character, has layers of rock running in a perpendicular direction, with their edges projecting in vast shelves.

In different parts also are projections interspersed with patches of verdure, samphire, &c. in the most romantic stile. The top of the highest part, where it is the most easy of access, is about two or three yards wide, but as it advances towards the arch, it becomes much more contracted. When on the top, a tremendous precipice strikes the mind with horror, its perpendicular height being about 180 feet. Through this arch boats frequently sail.

Lulworth Cove is a fine natural curiosity. It forms a snug circular harbour, in which vessels of eighty tons may ride with security. It appears as if scooped out of the rock, and is surrounded by lofty cliffs, except towards its entrance from the sea.

Sailing and fishing in the bay is a frequent and pleasant amusement at Weymouth, and for this every facility is furnished by the industrious and obliging boatmen of the place.

RIDES ROUND WEYMOUTH.

PORTLAND.

Portland, about four miles from Weymouth, is commonly called an island, but is, properly speaking, a peninsula, as it joins the main land by an isthmus, composed of a ridge of pebbles.

The nearest way from Weymouth is to be ferried over an inlet of the sea at the end of Smallmouth sands, for which the following rates are paid: Foot-passengers each, 1*d.* with a horse, 2*d.* single chaise, 1*s.* 6*d.* post-chaise, 2*s.* 6*d.* coach, 3*s.* 6*d.*

On the Portland side of the ferry the beach or ridge of pebbles is worthy the attention of every visitant, who will be astonished to find a loose pebbly shore, extending from Portland to Abbotsbury, a space of more than nine miles, capable of resisting the most furious tempests. The pebbles, contiguous to Portland, are nearly the size of an egg, but they gradually diminish, till they are lost in fine gravel. Many of them are beautifully veined, and others quite transparent, and capable of being converted into seals and other trinkets.

That inlet of the sea which runs by the passage-house, for the space of five miles, is called the fleet. On its borders is a seat belonging to Mr. Gould of Upway.

Approaching Portland, the castle appears on the left, which, with that on the opposite shore of Weymouth, was built in the reign of Henry VIII. when he made a general fortification of the coasts.

The tour of Portland generally commences at the top of the hill, where, in a little hut, one of the quarrymen exposes for sale specimens of the various productions of the island, consisting of spar, fossils, ores, shells, &c. On both sides of this summit may be seen some of the immense quarries from which that beautiful and durable stone is taken, that has been used in building some of the most magnificent edifices in this country.

The New Light-house, built by the late Mr. Johns, of Weymouth, is a well-adapted conical edifice, sixty-three feet high, containing inside a geometrical staircase, by which there is an easy ascent to the top, where a curious apparatus is fixed for the lights which direct the hardy sons of Neptune, through the dangerous navigation of Portland Race.

From hence, on a clear day, may be seen Torbay on the right, and the Isle of Wight on the left, at the distance of twenty-five leagues.

Near this edifice is the signal-house, and not far off is Cave's Hole, a large cavern perforated by the sea, a great way into the rocks, having an aperture on the land through which the foaming element may be seen and heard, in all its terrors.

On the southern part of Portland may be viewed the remains of Bow-and-Arrow Castle, and near this are the ruins of the old church, which, though now close to the cliff, was formerly said to have stood in the centre of the island. In this vicinity is a range of rocks, which appear to have been torn from the main body by some convulsive effort of nature, forming a chasm beautifully grand.

In Portland are two good houses of entertainment; the first stands at the entrance of Chiswell, and is called the New Hotel; the other at Fortune's

Well,* and is known by the sign of the Portland Arms. These houses meet with great encouragement; for scarcely a person comes to Weymouth who does not devote a day at least to visit the romantic scenery of Portland, which contains seven villages, Chissel, Fortune's Wells, Rayfourne, Wakeham, West Town, East Town, and South Well.

The inhabitants, amounting to about 2000, who are chiefly employed in the quarries, are a robust and hardy race. They were formerly famous for slinging of stones, and were the ancient Baleares of Britain.

They are a honest simple people, and their integrity has become proverbial. "On the word of a Portland man" is esteemed a high sanction in contracts and engagements. They have some particular customs of their own, to which they adhere with inviolable constancy. It is said that the young men and women cohabit together before marriage, and if no signs of fruitfulness appear in due time, they part, and look out for other mates, not thinking they were designed by providence for each other.

On the summit of the hill, behind the Portland Arms,† are some traces of a Roman encampment.—The quarries, however, and the manner in which they are worked, are the most curious objects in this insulated spot.

ABBOTSBURY.

This inelegant town, distant about eight miles from Weymouth, receives its appellation from its an-

* Fortune's Well is a fine and never-failing spring, which rises at the height of more than 200 feet above the level of the sea.

† The landlord of the Portland Arms usually has it in his power to shew the Reevepole, or Saxon mode of keeping accounts, and by which the bailiff of the island collects the manor dues, as on this pole every acre of land within its limits is described.

cient abbey, founded by Orcus, steward of the household to King Canute. It appears to have occupied a large space of ground. In the vicinity is St. Catherine's Chapel, a curious remnant of antiquity, which, standing on a high hill, serves as a sea-mark. Here also are several druidical monuments, consisting of temples and altars.

The swannery and decoy for wild ducks in this neighbourhood, likewise engage the attention of the inquisitive.

DORCHESTER.

Dorchester, the county town, situate about eight miles from Weymouth, is a place of great antiquity, having been a principal station both in the Roman and Saxon times. The castle stood on the spot now occupied by a county goal, on an eminence, at the foot of which flows the river Froome.

This town is remarkable for the amenity of its situation, and the extensive downs in its vicinage, which produce the sweetest herbage, and give a peculiarly fine flavour to the mutton.

About half a mile from Dorchester, on the right, lies Manbury, a complete Roman amphitheatre, covering an acre of ground, in which 10,000 persons might have been accommodated.

On the road to Dorchester lies the village of Monckton, containing two or three gentlemen's seats, and immediately behind it stands Maiden Castle, one of the most perfect remains of ancient fortification in this kingdom. It is of an oval form, containing an area of between forty and fifty acres, surrounded by a treble ditch, and ramparts of great depth and length, From hence is an expansive view of the country, taking some of the hills in the Isle of Wight. A great number of barrows are seen in the environs of Maiden Castle.

LULWORTH CASTLE.

About sixteen miles from Weymouth stands Lulworth castle, which, notwithstanding its distance from Weymouth, is a constant object of attraction to strangers. It is the seat of Thomas Weld, esq. and is not only admired for its situation, but in itself forms a most superb pile, adorned with statuary, paintings, fine gardens, and other elegant and beautiful accompaniments. The environs are extremely well wooded, and happily intersected by hill and dale.—From the south front of the house is seen a beautiful expanse of water, and a moving scene of ships.

Lulworth probably retains the name of Castle, from its being built on the site of an ancient fortress. The present edifice was erected about 1600. The possessor being of the Roman Catholic persuasion, has fitted up a beautiful chapel, and made many other improvements in his mansion and domain.

The magnificent manner in which Mr. Weld received their majesties and the royal family, when they did him the honour of a visit some years ago, would reflect a lustre on the taste, opulence, and loyalty, of the first subject in the kingdom.

The pictures and other works of art are too numerous to particularize, but they may be seen every Wednesday, from ten to two.

Other places more distant, such as Sherborne, Blandford, Corfe Castle, Wareham, and Cerne Abbey, are occasionally visited by company, who make Weymouth their summer residence; and in its immediate vicinity are several favourite spots, which, however, in a more fertile and picturesque country, would be wholly overlooked. The same may be said of some seats in the environs of Weymouth, which are only remarkable because there is little opportunity of comparing and contrasting them. Yet, independent of local considerations, that shore must be dear to Britons, from whence their monarch, wearied with the toils of state, has often returned in renovated health and spirits.—Long may Weymouth be honoured with his summer visit, and may its tides and its breezes waft to him and the partner of his throne, all their salutary influences!

WORTHING.

WORTHING, distant fifty-nine miles from London, and eleven westward of Brighton, possesses many attractions, which contribute to render it a desirable residence for those who wish to enjoy the benefits of air or sea-bathing. It is surrounded, at the distance of not quite a mile, by the uninterrupted chain of the Sussex Downs, which, forming nearly an amphitheatre, completely exclude, even in the winter months, the chilling blasts of the north and east winds. It is a common thing to see a considerable number of bathers here, even in the depth of winter, the thermometer being generally higher than at Brighton, and on an average, between two and three degrees above what it is at London. Besides, this rural village possesses other powerful recommendations; a facility of bathing, in the most stormy weather, and an extent of sand, as level as a carpet, of at least seven miles towards the west, and three to the east, on which the pedestrian or the horseman may enjoy the full refreshment of the sea breeze, during the reflux of the tide, without interruption.

Never was there an instance of the effects of public partiality more strongly exemplified than at Worthing. In a short space of time, a few miserable fishing huts and smugglers' dens have been exchanged for buildings sufficiently extensive and elegant to accommodate the first families in the kingdom. The establishment of two respectable libraries, (Spooner's and Stafford's) at each of which the newspapers are regularly received, and the erection of commodious warm baths (Wickes's) within a few years; sufficiently prove how far it has risen in public estimation.

Worthing is in the parish of Broadwater, a village about the distance of half a mile, which now looks contemptible when contrasted with the growing splendour of its dependent.

The manor of Broadwater formerly belonged to the family of the Camois, who flourished from the time of Edward the first till the sixteenth century. A singular anecdote is recorded of sir John Camois, who by a deed regularly executed, "of his own free will, gave and demised *his wife Margaret* to sir William Painel, knight, with all her goods, chattels, and other appendages, to have and to hold during the term of her natural life." This instance of packing off a wife, bag and baggage, shews that Pope Gregory was not mistaken when he wrote to Lanfranc, archbishop of Canterbury, that he had heard there were certain persons in Scotland, who not only forsook, but sold their wives, whereas in England they gave and granted them away.

The neighbourhood of Worthing is exceeded by no place in the kingdom, in the variety and agreeableness of its rides. The downs are always dry, the soil being chalky, with brown mould or clay, and, where cultivated, produce good crops of corn, besides feeding large flocks of sheep.

The modern buildings of Worthing are immediately upon the coast, but the village extends towards the downs in a straight line for about half a mile. The inhabitants entertain apprehensions from the inroads of the sea, which, as they say, has been progressively gaining ground for the last thirty years, and some even recollect when houses stood where the sea now flows.

The manor of Broadwater lately belonged to the earl of Warwick, who built a very noble house at Worthing, fronting the sea, the last owner of which was major Commerell, of the Life Guards.

Among the conveniences of Worthing must not be omitted the facility with which visitors are at all times accommodated with good saddle-horses, if they do not come already provided for country exercise.

The post arrives about ten o'clock, and leaves Worthing again about three.

The villages in the vicinity of this place have been described in the accounts of Brighton, Bognor, and Little Hampton.

The visitor at Worthing will find his interest in the beauties of this place considerably increased, by the perusal of A Tour to Worthing, written by the liberal and ingenious author of the Sketch of Religious Denominations, and of various other useful works, by the rev. J. Evans, M.A.

YARMOUTH.

As a sea-bathing place, Yarmouth possesses some advantages over its more fashionable rivals. From the great extent of the town, lodgings are numerous, and comparatively reasonable, and provisions are not only plentiful but cheap. To those, therefore, who study economy, Yarmouth presents powerful attractions, particularly when the local circumstances of the party are favourable for making it a bathing visit.

SITUATION, HISTORY, TRADE, &c.

Yarmouth, distant about 124 miles from London, and twenty-two from Norwich, stands on a peninsula, at the eastern extremity of the county of Norfolk, encompassed on the south and east by the sea, on the north by the main land, and on the west by the Yare, over which is a handsome draw-bridge, connecting it with Suffolk. It extends rather more than a mile in length, and nearly half a mile in breadth, containing four principal streets, running from north to south, and 156 narrow lanes, or rows, intersecting them in the opposite direction. It is surrounded by a wall, with ten gates and sixteen towers, on the east, north, and south sides; and according to the parliamentary enumeration of 1801, has a population of nearly 15,000 souls.

Yarmouth is an ancient borough-town, governed by a mayor, aldermen, and other officers, and has sent representatives to parliament ever since Edward I. The number of electors, consisting of freemen by inheritance, servitude, or purchase, is about 800. The corporation possesses extensive privileges.

The markets, on Wednesdays and Saturdays, are plentifully supplied; the houses are well built, and respectably tenanted; and, among the polite amusements of the place, may be reckoned the Theatre, the Assembly-room, and Concerts, during the bathing-season. A considerable fishery is carried on here, which, with its foreign trade, throws a constant animation over the shore; and such as are fond of aquatic excursions, fishing, shooting, bowling, and other manly diversions, may find ample opportunity of gratifying their inclinations at Yarmouth.

The situation of this town is favourable for commerce; and, besides fishing-vessels, which are numerous, upwards of 300 ships belong to the port, which trade to Holland, France, Norway, and the Baltic, or carry on a coasting traffic.

Among the peculiarities of this place is the general use of a low narrow cart, well adapted to the confined rows, or lanes, through which it must pass. It is drawn by a single horse, and is much employed in conveying goods to and from the shipping. Others, more elegantly made, which go by the name of Yarmouth coaches, are let for airings to the fort, along the downs, or to other places in the environs. Every stranger makes a point of being drawn in one of these vehicles, by way of amusement; or, at least, to have the credit of riding in one of the most whimsical carriages known in this kingdom. On sandy roads, however, which abound here, they sink so deep as to look like sledges drawing traitors to the place of execution; and on the rough pavement of the town, the nerves must be very strong to endure the motion.

THE QUAY.

The entire length of the quay is upwards of a mile and a furlong, and, in some places, it is 150 yards wide. From the bridge to the south gate it is decorated with a fine range of buildings, among which the assembly-house makes a conspicuous figure. The quay forms a fashionable and delightful promenade, and is maintained at a great expence.

MARKET-PLACE.

The market-place forms a handsome area; but, to

render it pleasant for visitors, the butchers ought to be under better regulations, and several nuisances should be removed. The sight of animals slaughtered must offend the delicate, and wound the feelings of the humane.

THE THEATRE.

This edifice, which was erected in 1778, is neat, and well-adapted to its destination. It occupies the site of a chapel formerly belonging to the Dutch congregation. The Norwich company of comedians, under the management of Mr. Brunton, perform here a certain number of weeks in winter, and part of the summer. They justly rank next to those of London, Bath, and York.

ASSEMBLY-ROOM, &c.

The assembly-room is not of the first order of elegance, but it perfectly answers the purpose. We have frequently seen more cheerful countenances in a barn than in the finest ball-room in the kingdom. Assemblies are held here every week, during the bathing season. Amusements of every kind are to be purchased, on easy terms, at Yarmouth. The bowling-green, on the east bank of the river, is pleasantly situated, and well attended.

THE BATH-HOUSE.

This building, which was erected in 1759, cost nearly 1000*l.* It stands on the beach, which is a sinking sand, about three furlongs distance from St. George's chapel. The vestibule is a neat, well-proportioned room, with windows fronting the town and the sea. On the right of the entrance are four closets, having each a door into the bath-room. This bath is fifteen feet by eight, and is appropriated for gentlemen. A similar one is assigned for the use of the ladies.

The marine fluid is raised every tide, by a horse-mill, into a reservoir, at the distance of fifty yards from the baths, into which it is conveyed by separate pipes. In short, the accommodations here are perfectly adapted either to the bather for health, or for pleasure: the attendance is good, and the charges are reasonable.

As for the machines, they are sufficiently commodious; but, as they stand at a distance from the town, it is not very pleasant to ride on sand up to the horse's belly, or to walk in it up to the knees.

Adjoining to the north end of the Bath-house, a large and pleasant public room was built, in 1788, where company are accommodated with tea and coffee, morning and afternoon; a public breakfast, on Tuesdays and Fridays; and occasional concerts, during the season. Here the London and country newspapers are provided; and, as there is no coffee-room in the town, this may be said to be the most fashionable and agreeable lounge. The subscription is 5*s.* for a gentleman, and 2*s.* 6*d.* for a lady, for the room and the papers. Tea, coffee, and concerts, are equally reasonable.

The jetty, close to the Bath-house, is 110 paces long, and 24 feet broad at the head. This forms an agreeable walk after bathing; and the lively scene of ships, almost perpetually under sail, in various directions, tends to dissipate that ennui which is apt to creep on those who have been accustomed to active employments.

THE CHURCH.

The church, dedicated to St. Nicholas, the patron of fishermen, is a large and stately pile, about 250 feet long, and including the aisles, 108 in breadth. The spire, which appears crooked in every direction, is 186 feet high, and serves for a sea-mark at a great distance. The sailors, who are in the habit of passing Yarmouth, when they see this twisted spire, jocularly observe, that there never was but one virtuous woman married in this church, and that the spire, out of compliment, made a bow to her, and has ever since retained its bending posture. In the church is an excellent organ.*

St. Nicholas was the only place of worship, of the establishment, in this populous place, till 1717, when a beautiful chapel was built near the centre of the town, and dedicated to St. George.

INNS, COACHES, &C.

The Angel, and Wrestlers, are excellent houses of entertainment, and lodgings may be hired in most parts of the town, but the market-place is preferred. The mail arrives every day from London; and there is no want of conveyances between this place and the metropolis, as well as the neighbouring towns. A barge sails twice a week to Norwich, in which there are good accommodations for passengers.

Though Yarmouth Roads, on the east side of the town, are the chief rendezvous of colliers and merchantmen passing and re-passing in this direction, yet the shore is one of the most dangerous to mariners of any on the coast of Britain, many melancholy instances of which are recorded. In 1692, 200 sail of ships, and upwards of 1000 people, were lost in one night; and a somewhat similar misfortune happened in 1790.

RIDES AND WALKS ROUND YARMOUTH.

The sea-coast of Yarmouth, for about two miles each way, is nearly a level common, elevated two or three yards above high-water mark. From the verdant edge of this common to the sea is a gentle slope, composed of deep sand, intermixed with shingle. Along this beach, particularly to the southward of the town, the botanist will find the bunias cakile, or sea rocket, the salsolà kali, or prickly glasswort; the arundo arenaria, or sea-reed grass, or marrum; the arenaria peploides, or sea-chick-

* The first mention of organs, in this part of Europe, is of one which Constantine Capronimus, emperor of the east, sent to Pepin, king of France, about the year 757.

weed; the eryngium maritimum, or sea-holly; the convolvulus soldanella, or sea-bird weed; the ononis repens, or creeping rest-harrow; and several other marine plants; which render a walk along this spot pleasant and amusing.

CAISTER.

About two miles from Yarmouth are the ruins of Caister, the ancient seat of the family of Falstolff, which, however, have no affinity to the fat Knight of Shakespeare; as Sir John Falstolff, who built the castellated mansion of Caister, was one of the most valiant generals, and respectable men, of his age. The remains of this edifice shew it to have been capacious and strong, and it well deserves a visit from the inquisitive.

From the coins, and other remains of antiquity, which are occasionally dug up in this vicinity, it is evident the Romans had a station here as well as at

BURGH CASTLE,

Which stands on the opposite side of the river, in the county of Suffolk. Possessing an elevated situation, it commands an extensive view of the road and coast, and seems to have been admirably calculated, both for alarm and defence. The walls, composed of rows of brick and flint alternately, are nine feet thick, and fourteen feet high, inclosing an area of four acres and a half. On the east side, which is most perfect, are the remains of four flanking towers.

The country, from Caister to Burgh Castle, is a continued plain of three miles in length, the greatest part of which, if we may believe tradition, was once covered with water.

APPENDIX.

OUTLINE
OF A
TOUR OF THE LAKES,
IN
Cumberland, Westmoreland, and Lancashire.

AS numerous parties and individuals every season, actuated by the pursuit either of health or pleasure, visit the LAKES, or make a partial or general TOUR of WALES, in order to render this *vade mecum* more complete, brief accounts of both are appended, not so much indeed with a view of gratifying curiosity, as of exciting it. To the Tours of the Lakes and of Wales, already published, it is almost impossible to add any thing new, nor is it the object of this work to enter into details,

"Where pure description holds the place of sense,"

but to direct the inquisitive, and to furnish useful information to the stranger.

West, who has long been considered as the legitimate guide to the LAKES, adapting his work for those who approach them by the way of Lancaster, describes them in the subsequent order: CONISTON, ESTHWAITE, WINDERMERE, RYDAL, GRASMERE, LEATHES, DERWENT, BUTTERMERE, CRUMMOCK, LOWES, ULLS, and HAWS, and from him we borrow the following Itinerary.

From LANCASTER to the LAKES.

Miles.		Miles.	
	LANCASTER.	2	Holker-gate.
3	Hest-bank.	3	Over Ulverston-sands to Carter-House.
9	Over Lancaster sands to Carter-House.	1	ULVERSTON.
2	Cartmel church town, or Hookburgh.	12	Dalton, Furness Abbey and back to Ulverston

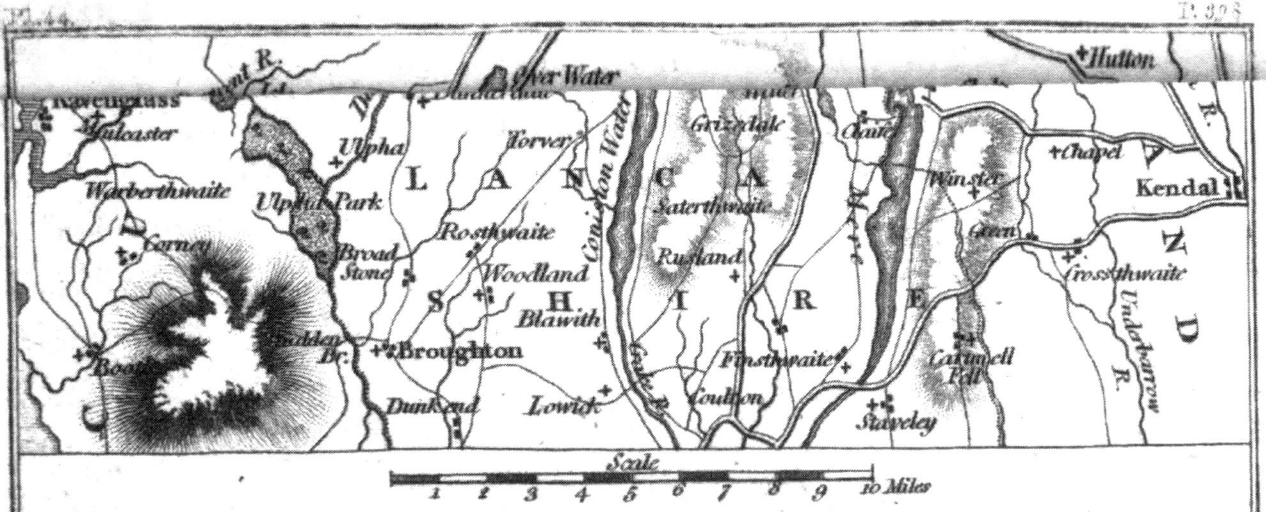

Pl. 44.
P. 323
Hutton
Over Water
Walcaster
Warberthwaite
Corney
Ulpha
Ulpha Park
Broad Stone
Duddon Br.
Broughton
Dunkend
Torver
Rosthwaite
Woodland
Blawith
Lowick
Coniston Water
Grizedale
Saterthwaite
Rusland
Finsthwaite
Coulton
Winster
Cartmell Fell
Staveley
Chapel
Kendal
Crossthwaite
Underbarrow R.
L A N C A S H I R E
A N D
Scale
1 2 3 4 5 6 7 8 9 10 Miles

THE LAKES

Miles.
4 Penny-Bridge.
2 Lowick-Bridge, or
5 From Ulverston to Lowick-Bridge.
2½ Through Nibthwaite to Coniston Waterfoot.
6 **Coniston** Waterhead.
3 Hawkeshead.
5 To **Ambleside.**
2 **Rydal.**
2 **Grasmere.**
2½ Dunmail-raise-stones.
3¼ Dalehead.
4¼ Castle-rigg.
1 **Keswick.**
3 **Lowdore** Waterfall.
1 Grange.
1 Bowdar-Stone, Castle-Hill.
2¼ Rosthwaite.
2½ Seathwaite.
9 Keswick.
8 Down Bassenthwaite-water by Bowness, Bradness, Scareness, to Armathwaite.
9 Up the other side of the Lake to Keswick.
5 Gasgadale.
3 **Buttermere.**
6 Down Crummock-water to Lorton.

Miles.
7½ Keswick.
4 Threlkeld.
6 Whitbarrow.
1 Penruddock.
6¼ **Penrith.**
5 Dunmallet, at the foot of Ulls-water, and Pooly-Bridge.
9 Water Millock, Gowbarrow-Park, Airy-Bridge, to the head of Ulls-water.
9 Ambleside, or
14 To Penrith.
10½ By Lowther, Askham, and Brampton, to Haws-water.
15 From the head of Haws-water through Long-Sleddale, to Kendal; or
5 To Shap, by Rosgill and Shap Abbey.
7 Hawse-foot.
8 **Kendal.**
10 Down the east side of Kent to Levens-Park, and return to Kendal by Sizergh.
11 Burton in Kendal.
11 **Lancaster.**

Mr. Housman, whose "Descriptive Tour of the Lakes," &c. is a real acquisition to British Topography, taking up the stranger at Kendal or Penrith, recommends the Lakes to be visited in the following succession: **Haws**, **Ulls**, **Derwent**, **Bassenthwaite**, **Buttermere**, **Crummock**, **Lowes**, **Ennerdale**, **Wast**, and returning to **Keswick**, from thence to **Leathes**, **Grasmere**, **Rydal**, **Windermere**, **Esthwaite**, and **Coniston**.*

* "Tourists from Scotland," says Mr. Housman, "will find it most convenient to proceed from Carlisle to Ousebridge, at the lower end of Bassenthwaite-water. After visiting that Lake, they may either go directly to Kendal,

We take the liberty to select that part of Mr. Housman's route which is connected with the Lakes, and notice them in the order he has indicated, leaving our readers to follow him or Mr. West, according to their fancies, or to the circumstances or situation in which they are placed, when they commence their tour.

From Kendal through the Lakes to Lancaster.

Miles.		*Miles.*	
	KENDAL.	2¼	Seathwaite.
15	Haws-water, through Long Sleddale.	4½	Wast-water, over Stye-head.
12	PENRITH, by Brampton and Lowther.	13¼	KESWICK, by Watenlath
5	ULLSWATER-FOOT.	8	Armthwaite, down the east side of Bassenthwaite-water.
9	Patterdale, or head of Ullswater.	9	Keswick, up the other side.
9	AMBLESIDE, over Kirkstone.	5	Keskadale.
15	KESWICK, from Ullswater.	3	BUTTERMERE.
3	Lodore-water-fall.	1½	Scale-force.
1	Grange.	6	Lorton, from Buttermere, down Crummock water.
1	Bowdar-stone, Castle-hill.	7½	Keswick.
1	Rosthwaite.	1	Castle-rigg.

or first visit Buttermere, and the adjacent Lakes. From Keswick proceed to Ambleside; and having viewed the beauties of Windermere, cross the ferry to Coniston, by way of Hawkeshead. From thence the traveller might ride to Kendal by way of Newby-bridge, or pursue his route still further to Ulverston and Furness, and after visiting the antiquities there, enjoy the pleasure of a new scene, in a journey from Ulverston to Lancaster, over the sands. Return from Lancaster by Kendal, Haws-water, Ulls-water, and Penrith, to Carlisle.

"The caves in Yorkshire may be visited either before or after the Lakes, as it may suit the convenience or inclination of the tourist;" or they may be wholly omitted, by which very little will be lost, except to persons of a particular taste. "What is the cave remarkable for?" said the ingenious and elegant Mr. Grant to a countryman who accompanied him. "It is remarkable," replied he, "for being a nasty, damp place, with a mortal deal of water in it." The same character will apply to the generality of the Yorkshire caverns.

Page 475

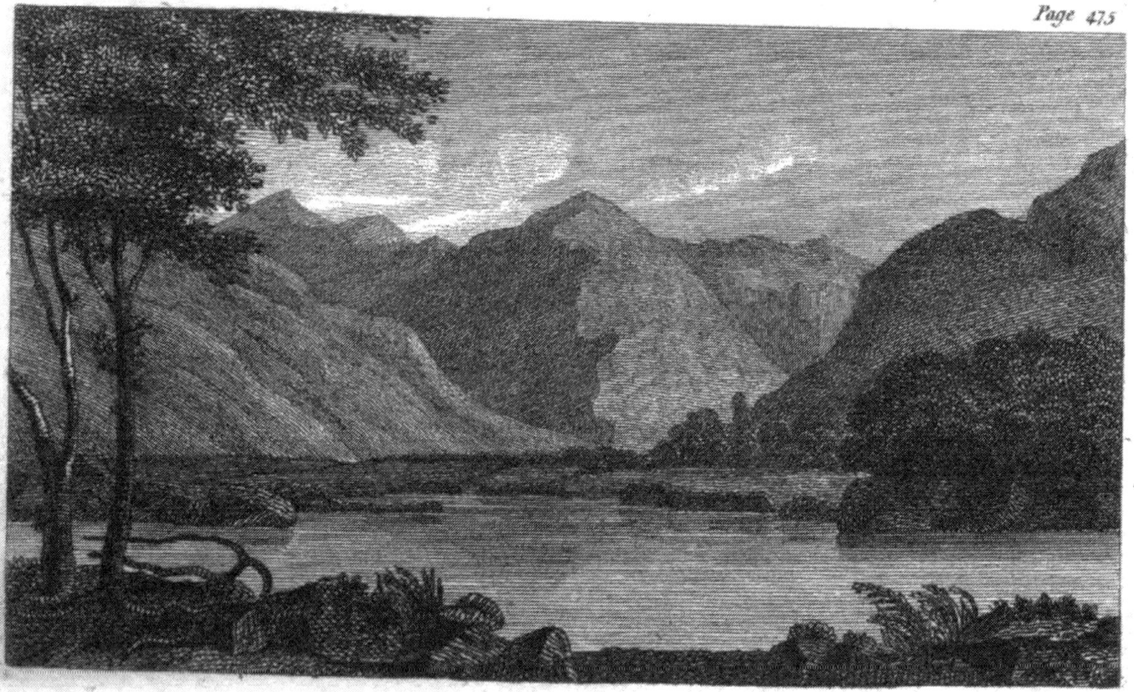

Ullswater.

Miles.		Miles.	
4	LEATHES-WATER.	4	Levens.
4½	Dunmaile-raise-stones.	2	Milnthorp.
2½	GRASMERE.	4	Burton.
2	RYDAL.	7	Bolton.
2	AMBLESIDE.	4	LANCASTER.
6	Bowness.	5	ULVERSTON from Lowick-Bridge.
1	Ferry-house, across Windermere.	6	Furness Abbey, by Dalton.
4	Hawkeshead.	1	Carter-House, from Ulverston.
3	CONISTON-WATER-HEAD.	3	Holker.
6	Coniston-water-foot.	2	Cartmel or Flookburgh
2½	Lowick-Bridge.	2	Carter-House.
2	Penny-Bridge.	9	Hest-bank, over Sands.
2	Booth.	3	LANCASTER.
3	Newby-Bridge.		
3	Newton.		
4	Witherslack.		

HAWS (OR HALLS) WATER.

The approach to this lake, which is an easy and pleasant morning ride from Penrith, is very picturesque. You pass between two high ridges of mountains, the banks finely spread with enclosures. The lake is about three miles long, and half a mile at the broadest part, almost divided in the middle by a promontory of enclosures, joined by a strait. The features of the two divisions are different, and this adds to the beauty of each. The narrowest part is reported to be 50 fathoms deep, and a man may throw a stone across it. Char, perch, trout, eel, and other fish, are caught here.

ULLS-WATER.

This lake lies about five miles south-west from Penrith, by a most delightful road. Ulls-water is of great length, though seldom more than three quarters of a mile in breadth. After extending itself about 3½ miles in a line to the south-west, it bends at the foot of Place-fell almost due west, and is soon again interrupted by the foot of Helvellyn, a lofty and very rugged mountain; and spreading again, turns off to the south-east, and is lost among the deep recesses of the hills. Its whole length cannot be less than nine miles. The scenery on its banks is of the first order for picturesque effect. Near the head of the lake lies Patterdale, which has long given the local appellation of *king* to the Mounsey family, on account of their possessing the largest property in this sequestered spot.

DERWENT-WATER.

Derwent-water is about three miles long, and a mile and a half in the broadest part, forming an irregular figure. It stands near the little elegant town of KESWICK, and presents many features of exquisite beauty. The best method of viewing this enchanting lake is in a boat, or traversing its borders, round which there is an excellent road. Its bosom, transparent as crystal, is spotted with five beautiful sylvan islands, and the whole is guarded with mountains, among which Skiddaw towers in all its majesty. Several fine seats adorn the banks of Derwent-water. On the isle called formerly Vicar's island, is an elegant house belonging to the proprietor, Mr. Pocklington, whose name it now bears. The fall of Lodore is one of the principal beauties in the romantic vicinity of this beautiful lake, which is replete with every object that can delight or astonish.

BASSENTHWAITE-LAKE.

This lake is formed by the river Derwent, which serpentines through a delightful vale, after leaving the water of the same name. Bassenthwaite is nearly four miles long, and in some places expands to almost a mile in breadth. Its banks are agreeably varied with cultivation, and abrupt precipices which sometimes range with the water edge. In a word, the scenery would be esteemed exquisite, did it not lie so near the superior grandeur of Derwent-water.

BUTTERMERE.

Hail! awful scenes, that calm the troubled breast,
And woo the weary to profound repose,
Can passion's wildest uproar lay to rest,
And whisper comfort to the man of woes!
Here innocence may wander safe from foes,
And contemplation soar on seraph's wings.
O solitude! the man who thee foregoes,
When lucre lures him, or ambition stings,
Shall never know the source whence real grandeur springs.

So sings Beattie's Minstrel, Edwin, who it might be imagined, on contemplating the gloom, the grandeur, and the solitude of the environs of Buttermere, had this scene in his mind's eye. Yet even here it has been found *innocence* was not safe, and that *ambition* has led to ruin. The celebrated beauty of Buttermere, the daughter of the landlord of its rustic inn, will long be the object of pity and esteem, as she was formerly of admiration.

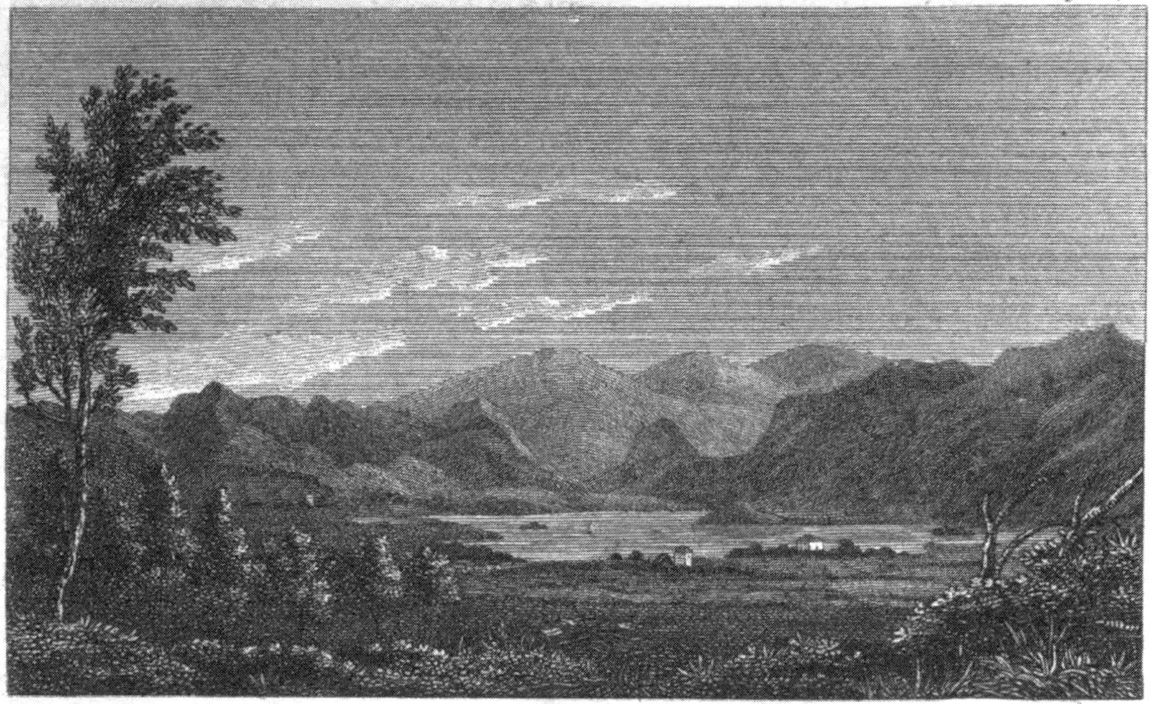

Derwentwater.

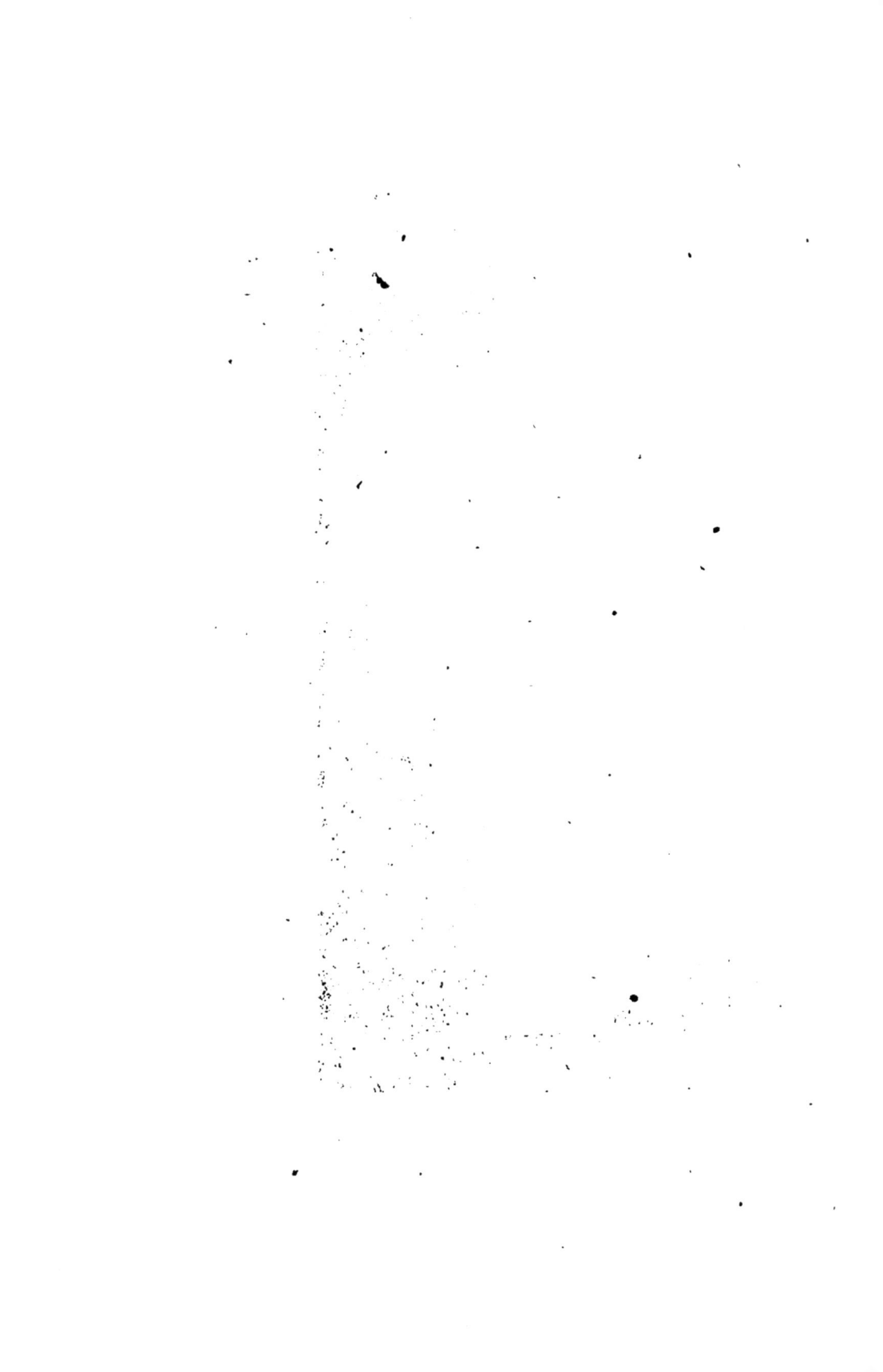

The little village of Buttermere stands on the eastern borders of a vale, as level as a bowling-green, and neatly divided into fields by quickset hedges. At each end of this plain a fine lake expands itself, stretching away to a great distance, amidst abrupt precipices and gently-sloping mountains. That in the south is called Buttermere, and that on the north Crummock-water. The former is a delightful sheet of water, about two miles long, and three quarters of a mile broad. Here pastoral life is seen in its original character.

CRUMMOCK-WATER.

The space between these two lakes is less than a mile, and consists of meadow and pasturage. This lake, which is about four miles long and half a mile in breadth, is adorned with three small isles, one of which is a naked rock, the others are covered with wood. There is a fine waterfall here, worthy the traveller's attention: and the surrounding scenery is exquisitely beautiful and romantic. Both Crummock and Buttermere are extremely deep and clear, and contain abundance of that delicate fish the char, which generally weighs from six to eight ounces, and is commonly sold by the dozen at 4s. 6d. The shores are sometimes wildly romantic and picturesque, and sometimes partake of the beautiful.

The chain of pyramidal mountains on each side of the narrow vale of Buttermere are highly picturesque. The river Cocker draws its supplies from Crummock-water.

LOWES-WATER.

This lake is about a mile in length, and almost uniformly about a quarter of a mile in breadth. The extremities are a charming mixture of woodland and cultivation, which rise up from the borders of the lake in waving lines; while lofty mountains bound the southern shore, that finely contrast with the softer features on the northern boundary.

Unlike the rest, Lowes-water has its course from north to south. The depth is not great, and it is destitute of char, but contains fine trout, and several other kinds of fish. It falls into Crummock-water under Mellbreack, and from this spot both lakes may be advantageously viewed.

ENNERDALE-WATER.

Between the last-mentioned lake and Ennerdale-water is an alpine pass over the wildest mountains of nearly four miles. This lake is so guarded indeed on all sides, except the west, by mountains almost inaccessible, that it is seldom visited in a general tour; but they who have a taste for mountain, sylvan, and pastoral scenery, will find it answer their expectation. It is about two miles and a half long, and three quarters of a mile broad in the widest part.

Before quitting the neighbourhood of Keswick, the traveller ought not to neglect visiting the museums of Crosthwaite and Hutton. The museum belonging to the former is a spacious building, and contains a profusion of singular curiosities collected in all parts of the world: that of the latter, who is a professed *ciceroni* to the lakes and mountains around, is likewise well filled with varieties, and antiques collected in his rambles. Being a practical botanist and mineralogist, his society is truly valuable to the lovers of natural history. At Keswick is a remarkable druidical monument or circle of stones, fifty in number. The traveller should also make an excursion by water as far as the bridge, in Borrowdale, as well for the pleasure of the romantic scenes as to visit the black-lead or wad-mines, which are opened only once in five years.

LEATHES-WATER, OR THIRLMERE-LAKE.

Proceeding towards Ambleside, come to Leathes-water, a narrow irregular sheet, which begins at the foot of Helvellyn, and skirts its base for the space of four miles, deriving considerable accessions from a variety of pastoral torrents, which devolve on the mountain's sides. On the right, Helvellyn and Catchidecam tower, in tremendous pomp. The opposite shore is bounded with crown-topp'd rocks of every aspect and form.

A remarkable beauty of this lake is, that it is almost intersected in the middle by two peninsulas, joined by a partial bridge, which seems intended as an easy communication for the shepherds that dwell on the opposite banks. Towards the farther extremity are two small islands agreeably clothed with wood; and at the termination of the lake is a pyramidal sylvan rock, which gives a charming finish to the scenery.

GRASMERE.

Passing Dunmaile-raise, a heap of stones, said to have been placed there to perpetuate the memory of the last King of Cumberland, we soon discover the sweetly sequestered vale of Grasmere, with its beautiful little lake, graced with a fine island, and bordered with some neat enclosures. This peaceful vale is about four miles in circumference, and is guarded by high mountains, among which Helm-cragg, at the upper end, presents a picturesque mass of antideluvian ruins. Nothing can be more beautiful than

Page 479

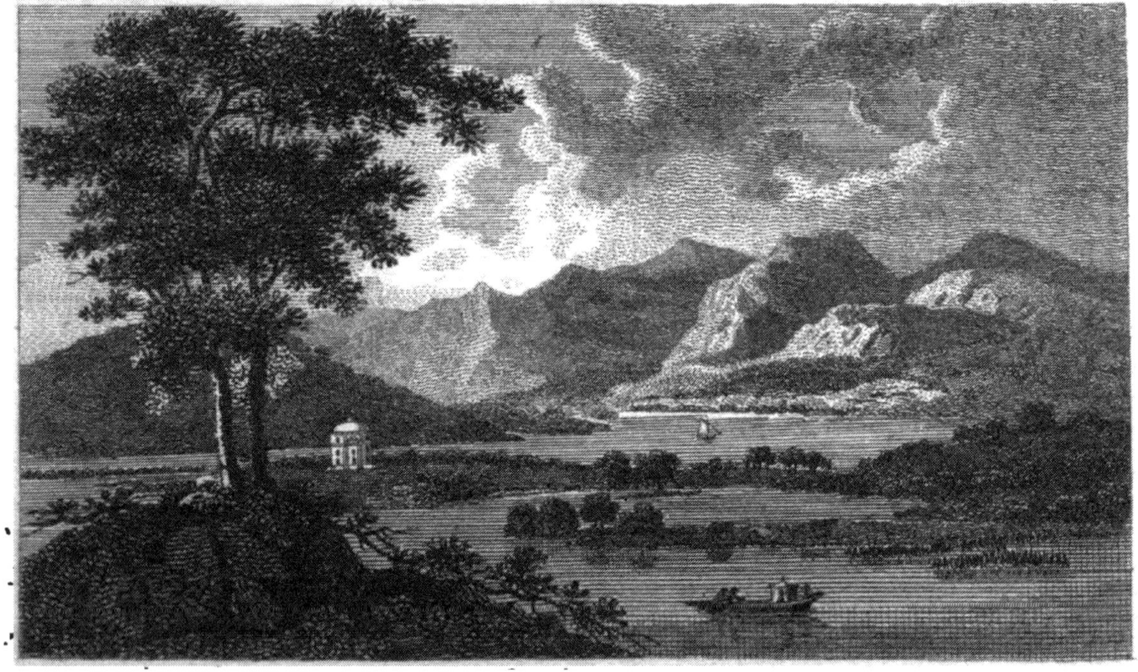

this lake and its accompaniments. Every part is in unison, and without the grandeur that arises from large extent, it is inexpressibly pleasing.

RYDAL-WATER.

This lake, which is about a mile long, and spotted with two little isles, communicates by a narrow channel with Grasmere, having the river Rothay for their common outlet. Some old woods grace its banks; and Rydall-hall, the seat of the late Sir Michael le Fleming, bart. situated on a gentle eminence, among waving woods, would be an ornament to any spot. There are two celebrated cascades, one at a little distance from the house in a sequestered glen, to which a convenient path conducts; the other is seen through the window of a summer-house, and, though small, it is beautiful beyond description.

WINDERMERE, OR WINANDERMERE.

This prince of the lakes is embosomed in a noble winding valley, about twelve miles long, every where enclosed with grounds, which rise in a very bold and various manner, in some places bursting into mountains, abrupt, wild, and uncultivated; in others breaking into rocks, craggy, pointed, and irregular; here rising into hills, covered with the noblest woods; there waving in glorious slopes of cultivated enclosures, enlivened with woods, villages, seats, and farms, scattered with picturesque confusion.

But what finishes the scene with an elegance too delicious to be imagined, is, that this noble expanse of water, which may vie with any thing in Britain, except Lough Lomond, is dotted with no less than ten islands, distinctly comprehended by the eye, from some points of view, all of the most bewitching beauty. Curwen's island, the largest, is of an oblong shape, swelling in the middle, and pointed at each end. It contains twenty-seven acres: and besides the neat mansion of its proprietor, John Christian Curwen, esq. it is laid out in the most enchanting style. Some of the other islets, called Holms, are also superbly robed. The lake is farther enlivened by a little fleet of vessels belonging to Mr. Curwen, and by Bowness, Lowood, Calgarth, and other places that adorn its banks.

The fish of Windermere are char, trout, perch, pike, and eel. The greatest depth of the lake is 222 feet, opposite to Ecclesrigg-cragg. The fall from Newby-bridge, where the current of the water becomes visible to the high-water mark of the tide at Lowood, distant two miles, is one hundred and five feet.

The principal feeders of this sublime and beautiful lake, are the rivers Rothay and Brathay, which unite their waters at the western angle of its head, and, after a short course, boldly enter this grand reservoir.

ESTHWAITE-WATER.

This lake is about two miles in length, and half a mile in breadth; and is almost cut in two by a peninsula, projecting on each side. These swelling projections are beautifully fringed with trees and coppice-wood, and cultivated at the top. The banks, which undulate regularly, are covered with soft verdure, cut in various fissures, with loose rows, intermixed with little groves and pendant woods, and have none of the romantic or rude features that form the barriers of most of the other lakes.

Near the head of Esthwaite is a small floating island, containing about two perches, covered with shrubs. Though connected with Windermere, no char have been found in this lake, probably because it wants a sufficient depth of water for this delicious species of fish.

CONISTON LAKE.

Of all the lakes, Coniston is most generally admired, and perhaps on just grounds. Its prevailing character is the romantic; and this character gives such scope to the imagination, that where it prevails, the beauty of the landscape must be supreme. A small island, covered with shrubs, rises in the middle of this charming lake, and adds to its picturesque effect.

Coniston is six miles long, and about one broad. Sequestered cottages are sprinkled on its banks, which form the base of craggy hills on the right and left. Below, they are verdant, with enclosures, and rich in woods, while the village of Coniston hanging half-way up, near a head-long torrent. The Black Beck of Torver encreases the general effect, to which Coniston-hall, a grey ivied mansion, essentially contributes. Above the verdant bordering the dark and rocky steps ascend to an alpine height, and encircle the head of the lake with a lofty amphitheatre. Copper mines are worked in the bowels of these mountains, which also produce abundance of blue slate.

Nothing can be more delightful than the navigation of Coniston, which exhibits almost all the varieties of scenery that are divided among the rest of the lakes. Nor is a ride round its shores less attractive, particularly under a morning sun, when all its beauties unfold themselves in full lustre.

Map catalogued

Pl. 48.

P. 412

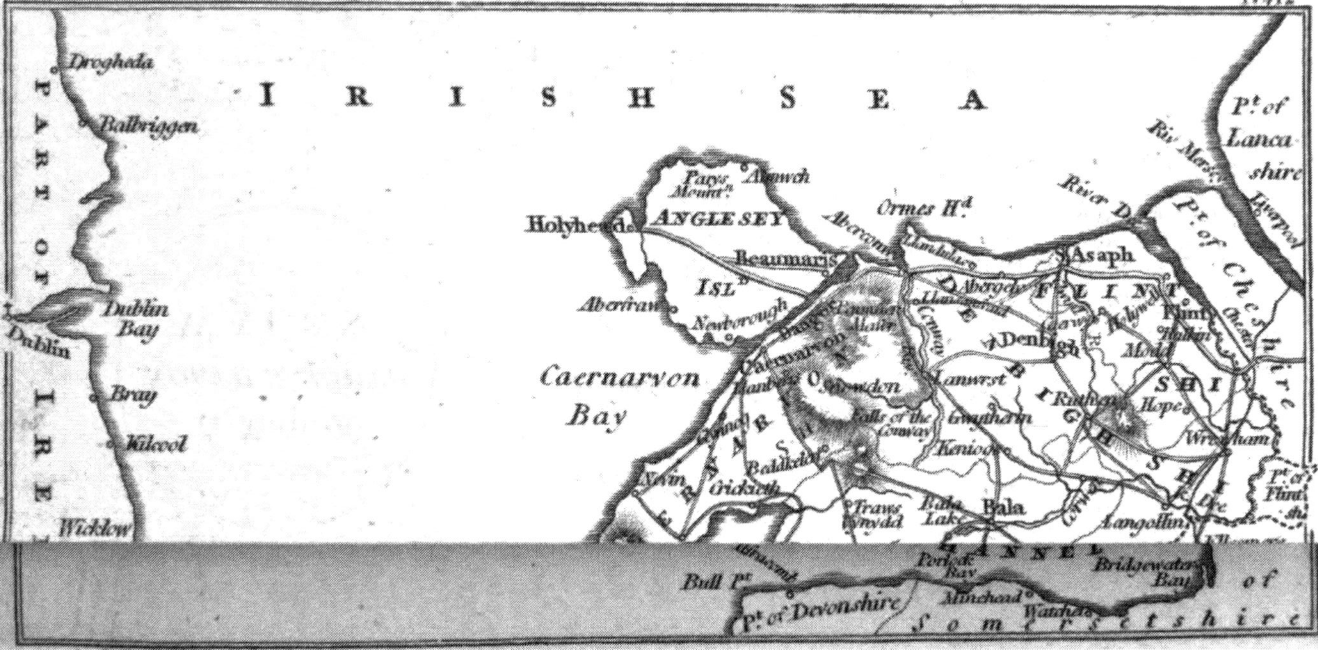
IRISH SEA
PART OF IRE
Droghada
Balbriggen
Dublin Bay
Dublin
Bray
Kilcool
Wicklow
Holyhead
ANGLESEY
Parys Mount
Amlwch
ISL
Beaumaris
Aberfraw
Newborough
Caernarvon Bay
Caernarvon
Snowden
Ormes Hd
Aberconway
Conway
Abergele
St Asaph
Denbigh
Lanwrst
Ruthin
Hope
Mold
Flint
Wrexham
Bala
Bala Lake
Trawsfynydd
Llangollin
Pt. of Cheshire
Chester
Liverpool
Riv Mersey
River Dee
Pt. of Lancashire
Pt. of Flint
Bridgewater Bay
Bull Pt.
Porlock Bay
Minehead
Watchet
Pt. of Devonshire
Somersetshire

In the words of Mr. Grant, we now sum up the characters of the principal lakes. "Windermere," observes he, "has that of immensity and variety of prospect, and we may add, of magnificence; Grasmere, of mildness; Derwent-water, of grandeur; but Coniston is elegant, and romantic, and sublime. We have since found the characters of the others—wildness of Crummock and Buttermere, and a combination of the whole in Ulls-water."

It will be satisfactory to those who feel an inclination to visit these romantic regions, to learn that the horses are sure-footed and easy, the guides civil, attentive, and sober, and the inns clean, comfortable, and reasonable.

SKETCH

OF A

TOUR IN SOUTH WALES.

Passing through the ancient city of Gloucester, cross the Severn, and proceed along its western bank to Newnham, where there is a ferry; and then deserting the banks of the river, travel through Mitchel-Dean to Ross, famous for being the birth-place of the benevolent Kyrle, immortalized by Pope, under the name of the Man of Ross.

Proceeding from thence by the navigation of the Wye, pass through Monmouth and Chepstow, both places of importance; and, after visiting the beautiful gardens of Piercefield, return to Chepstow, and making a digression, inspect the remains of the once-famous Caerwent, where is a curious tesselated pavement.

Crossing Penca Mawr, descend into the vale of Usk, and after visiting the town of the same name, proceed through Ragland, remarkable for its once-celebrated castle, the property of the Duke of Beaufort.

Reach the next town of Abergavenny, and from thence make an excursion to Llantony Abbey, part of which is still in tolerable preservation. From this sequestered spot, travel along an excellent road to Crickhowell, two miles and a half from which stands a stone called the county stone, to mark the entrance into Wales. The first house in the principality from this approach is called Sunny Bank. Pass through the village of Brolch to Brecknock where is a collegiate church, on the ruins of a benedictine priory.

Leaving Brecknock, pass through Merrthyr Tydvil, and crossing the Taaffe by the celebrated Pont-y-prydd, or New Bridge, proceed to Caerphilly, remarkable for its castle, the work of Edward I. one of the towers of which has long declined eleven feet from the perpendicular, and yet remains entire.

Pass through Pontipool and the ancient Caerlon to Cardiff, the capital of Glamorganshire, and one of the neatest towns of South Wales. Its old castle has been modernized, and is now the occasional residence of the Marquis of Bute, who is also Baron of Cardiff,

Directing our course towards Llandaff, an ancient episcopal see, now reduced to a village, pursue the road through Llantrissent, and from Cowbridge visit St. Donat's Castle, Pyle, Margam, and Aberavon.

Pursuing the course of the valley of Neath, inspect the mouldering remains of Neath Abbey, and then travel to Swansea,* which, for extent and beauty, exceeds all the towns of South Wales.

From Swansea, cross the country to Tenby,† and visit Pembroke, in whose castle Henry VII. was born. Reach Milford-Haven, capable of accommodating all the navies of Europe. Haberston Haiken, near its centre, forms the port; and at the extremity of one of the creeks stand the magnificent remains of Carew Castle.

Visit Picton Castle, the ancient seat of Lord Milford, five miles from which stands Haverfordwest, a large town, with a ruined castle.

Proceed over a dreary country to St. David's, which on account of its cathedral ranks as a city, though it is now a village, inhabited by fishermen. Here are some good houses, however, belonging to the ecclesiastical dignitaries. Make a diversion from thence to Fishguard, a miserable port; and, taking an inland direction, pass through the irregular town of Narberth to Carmarthen.

Carmarthen is a large and populous town, and boasts of very high antiquity, connected as well with classical history as with British superstition. Here the Romans had a station, and here the princes of South Wales formerly kept their court. It was once fortified, and had its castle situated on a rock commanding the River Towy, of which the gate only now remains converted into a county gaol.

Visit Dinevawr Park, and the proud ruins of its castle; view also at a distance, in the vale, Grongar-hill, immorta-

* See SWANSEA and its vicinity, described as a bathing-place.

† See also TENBY, as above.

lized by Dyer. After making a short stay at Llandilo, excurse to the cataract of Glen-kier and the ruins of Castle Caraigcennin, rising 400 feet perpendicular above the plain.

Reach Llanymdovery, a straggling town near the Upper Vale of Towy, bounded by a range of alpine hills, in which is the pass of Cwm-Dwr. Pursuing the road towards Builth, soon reach that beautifully situated place, on the banks of the romantic Wye, and thence make an excursion to Llandrindod Wells, about seven miles distant. This place, which is much frequented by the Welch gentry, possesses three different kinds of water; the rock water, the saline, and the sulphur water. The first is a chalybeate, strongly impregnated with iron, salt, and sulphur, and is recommended in nervous cases. The second is generally used for bathing, and when drank, is reckoned good in hypochondriac complaints. The third is used in scorbutic affections.

Passing through Llanymdovery, cross the Towy by a bridge of a single arch, and over a long range of steeps and declivities arrive at Newcastle, where the Tivy assumes the appearance of a river.

Directing our course to the sea-coast, reach the pleasant town of Cardigan, in whose vicinity stands Kilgarren, of which castle there are still some noble remains.

Taking the Aberystwith road, Cader Idris and many of the Merionethshire mountains open successively, and beguile the dreary path. The sea views, however, are very fine, and the country becomes more fertile towards Aberystwith.*

Having now reached the boundary of North Wales, take an eastern direction through the vale of Rhydol, and view, in advancing, the stupendous scenery of Cwm-Ystwith and Plinlimmon.

Cross the Monach by that singular edifice the Devil's Bridge: and visiting the beauties of Hafod, the seat of Mr. Johnes, pass through the wretched village of Cwm-Ystwith; and having gained the summit of the Cwmythen hills, obtain an uninterrupted retrospect of the dreary track behind.

Soon, however, a glorious prospect opens of the spacious plain through which the Wye flows, by the town of Rhyadergowy; at which place cross the Wye, by a bridge of a single arch, and proceeding towards Pen-y-bont, cross the Ithom, and pursue a rugged track over a wild range of hills, the scenes of many memorable exploits: and here the camp of Caractacus, and other antiquities, are still to be seen in high preservation.

---

* See ABERYSTWITH, and its vicinity, as a bathing-place.

Reach Presteign, the modern capital of Radnorshire; a place which, though much decayed, has still an air of neatness and comfort. Visit Old Radnor, which has now little to boast of, except its church. In the vicinity is that remarkable cataract called "Water-break-neck."

Again enter Builth, and proceed to Hay, a small market-town of Brecknock, remarkable for the ruins of its ancient castle.

Pass through the romantic village of Clyro, and here terminate the Tour of South Wales; in which the traveller at leisure will find numerous objects to interest and amuse.

It is almost a partiality unwarranted to point out any place in particular where these charms for the true lovers of nature may be discovered; so generally are they distributed throughout the principality. In truth, the diversified objects of pleasure, taste, genius, or simple curiosity, could not be exhausted either in this beautiful southern, or in the more sublime parts of the northern districts, which will be the subject of our next sketch; and so redundant are the sports of nature that solicit the feelings, engage the fancy, and luxuriate the eye, that with a slight change in the point of view, the same spot of ground might afford a painter a complete set of landscapes. Taken from the top of a mountain the valley might be sketched apart; and taken from the valley, a noble separate picture might be drawn of the mountain and its appropriate objects: join their several beauties by drawing them in a middle direction, the painter would soon feel how unnecessary it was to quit his native empire, to acquire the glory of his art.

SKETCH

OF A

TOUR IN NORTH WALES.

COMMENCING our Tour at Shrewsbury, the great frontier of England towards North Wales, make a digression to visit Hawkestone, late the Elysian residence of sir Richard Hill, though formed in the midst of a waste. Proceed from thence by Wemys to Oswestry, a handsome market-town on an eminence, crowned with the remains of a castle; and soon after, crossing the little river Cariac, enter the county of Denbigh.

Visit Chirk Castle, the noble seat of Mr. Middleton; cross the Dee to Wynnstay, the seat of sir Watkin Williams Wynne.

In the road to Wrexham, make a diversion to Erthig, the elegant mansion of Mr. Yorke. Offa's Dyke, not far from Wrexham, must not, on any account, be omitted in this rapid description of the Cambrian picture.—It was thrown up in the eighth century as a boundary between Mercia and the Britons, and extends from Basingwerk to Chepstow, in a line of 150 miles and upwards.

Soon after passing Wynnstay, a splendid mansion of sir Watkin Williams Wynne, an extensive well-wooded park, which is on the left of the road to Ruabon, we approach the interesting Llangollen, romantically situated in a vale environed with mountains, varied with woods, rocks, and torrents. On the summit of one of those mountains stand the ruins of Castle Dinas Bran, once inhabited by the beautiful Mifanwy Vechan, of whom the bard Hoel was deeply enamoured.

> Mid the gay towers in steep Din's Branna's cave,
> Her Hoel's breast the fair Mifanwy fires;
> O! harp of Cambria, never hast thou known
> Notes more mellifluent floating o'er the wires,
> Than when thy bard this brighter Laura sung,
> And with his ill-starr'd love Llangollen's echoe rung.
>
> Miss SEWARD.

"The fairy palace of the vale," the residence of the Right Hon. Lady E. Butler and Miss Ponsonby, whom an attachment as romantic as the situation they chose, but as beautiful to the affections, induced to quit the gay world, and retire to this sequestered spot, though the whole domain comprises little more than two acres, is picturesque and beautiful in the extreme, and has already rendered Llangollen a kind of classic ground, by the recording Muse of the elegant poet above quoted.

Passing from thence along a fine road, at the foot of the Berouin, enter the ancient and respectable city of Chester by a bridge over the Dee.

This being the frontier both towards North Wales and Ireland, has long been the principal approach to the former, and the grand thoroughfare to the latter. Proceed to Mold, in Flintshire, and visit Holywell, famous for St. Winifred's Well, which flows with such impetuosity, that its stream turns a number of copper, brass, and cotton mills, within a mile of its source. This well is still much frequented by Roman Catholics and others, and everal votive offerings of crutches still attest its triumphs over chronic diseases.

Take a view of the remains of Basingwerk Abbey; and, ascending a long and steep hill, enjoy a delightful prospect towards the coast, while, on the other hand, hill rises above hill in irregular confusion, till the Caernarvonshire mountains close the scene, with Snowden towering pre-eminent among them.

Descend into the fertile vale of Clwydd, watered by two little rivers; and, passing through Ruthyn, reach Denbigh, whose ancient castle is now no more than a picturesque ruin.

Crossing the Elvy, come to St. Asaph, the see of a Bishop; but remarkable for nothing, except its Gothic Cathedral.

Visit Abergely; and, winding round the mountain of Penmanross, catch a view of the magnificent ruins of Conway Castle, backed by the Caernarvonshire hills. Instead of directly crossing the ferry, proceed along the banks of the Conway to Llanrwst, remarkable for the amenity of its situation, and for its fine bridge.

Proceed a considerable way up the vale, and then, turning to the right, course the Llugwy to Pont-y-Pair. Penetrate into the recesses of the pile of mountains which forms the base of Snowden, to view the sublime cataract of Rhaidr-y-Wennel; and thence returning to Llanrwst, pass the old mansion of Gwydir.

Reach Conway, a picturesque object at a distance, but small, confined, and ill-built within. The castle, however, both for situation and extent, is one of the most magnificent ruins in Wales, and does honour to the taste and liberal spirit of Edward I.

Proceed towards the coast, and by the celebrated pass of Penmanmawr, reach the little town of Bangor, an episcopal see, peculiarly neat in its appearance, and agreeably situated in a vale, backed by the mountains.

Ferry over the Menai Straits to Anglesea, the ancient Mona, remarkable for its Druidical remains, and still more for its valuable mines of copper, which constitute its principal wealth. Beaumaris is the principal town, in the neighbourhood of which stands Baron Hill, the seat of lord Bulkeley.

Make an excursion to Holyhead, the great thoroughfare to Ireland, which has an excellent harbour. Next visit the Paris Mountain, whose copper-mine is upwards of a mile in circumference, and on an average employs 1300 men, in its various operations. The Mona and the Paris Lodge, belonging to the Earl of Uxbridge and Mr. Hughes, the two great proprietors of the mines, stand near the village of Amlwch.

Repass the Menai Straits at Bangor Ferry, and by an excellent road, commanding the most varied and majestic landscapes, reach Caernarvon, a neat and regular town, delightfully situated, and fashionably inhabited. In its castle the unfortunate Edward II., the first English Prince of Wales, was born.

Make an excursion to Pwlwhelli, Crickheith, and Penmorva, all miserable places, though agreeably situated; and, returning to Caernarvon, set out to explore the wonders of Snowden, whose head is frequently hid in clouds, and whose summit never can be gained without a guide. Take an advantageous view of this prince of mountains from Lake Llanberis, and, proceeding by the romantic pass of Beddgelert, enter the defile of the mountains, and soon see the cataract of Ys Gwyrfa, and in silent amazement contemplate the immense chains of surrounding mountains, among which Y Wyddfa, the lofty peak of Snowden towers, in all the pride of conscious superiority, over the vassal eminences.

After a night's repose at Caernarvon, having engaged an intelligent guide, set out to ascend Snowden, the highest hill in South Britain, its loftiest peak being 1300 yards above the level of the sea. The two first miles are rather boggy and disagreeable; but the remainder of the ascent, though more difficult and dangerous, is, in fine weather, recompensed by the prospects gradually opening, till on its summit, a plain of about six yards in circumference, the mind is lost in rapture and astonishment. From hence may be distinctly seen the Wicklow Hills, in Ireland, the Isle of Man, Cumberland, Lancashire, Cheshire, Shropshire, and part of Scotland, the Isle of Anglesea, and such a variety of objects more immediately under the eye, that a bare enumeration of them would be tedious.

> Thee, Snowden! King of Cambrian mountains, hail!
> With many a lengthen'd pause my lingering feet
> Follow the experienc'd guide; ———
> ——— while I gradual climb
> Thy craggy heights, through intermingled clouds,
> Various, of watery grey, and sable hue,
> Obscure the uncertain prospect from thy brow
> His wildest views the mountain Genius flings.
>
> SOTHEBY.

The easiest ascent of Snowden is from Dolbadarn Castle, in the vale of Llanberis, which a Welchman will take on one of his country's poneys. From hence, (says the Editor of the Cambrian Itinerary,) keeping on the side of a lake, turn to the left of Caunantmawr, a noble cataract; from thence ascend up a mountain to a vale called Cwm-Brwynog, a very deep and fertile spot, with little corn; but its principal produce are cattle and sheep. From here pass through Bwlch-y-Cwm Brwynog, where the ascent becomes so steep and difficult, that timid travellers are frequently obliged to clamber on foot among rocks, till, by keeping to the right, they arrive at Llyn-Glas. Llyn-Nadroedd, and Llynch-Coch, where the spaces between the precipices form a very agreeable isthmus, leading to a very verdant plain, where the traveller generally rests a short time. After this, a smooth path leads almost to the summit, called Y-Wyddfa, or the conspicuous, which rises to a point, leaving a small space for a circular wall of loose stones, within which travellers usually take their repast. The mountain from hence seems propped by four buttresses, between which are four deep curns, or valleys, with three lakes, and almost a boundless view.

Many who take this expedition set out during the night, on purpose to see the rising sun from the immense heights of Snowden; and, when the atmosphere is clear, no scene in nature can be more sublime than this, nor can the most glowing language paint it with effect.

The botanist and mineralogist will find abundant gratification in this ascent, as well as in that of Cader Idris. Alpine plants abound here: and the mineral substances which present themselves in succession, or lie blended together, are extremely various.

Storms, and fogs, and clouds, however, frequently surround the summit and sides of Snowden; and fortunate is that tourist who, at the first attempt, succeeds in ascending the Y-Wyddfa, and of finding the horizon propitious to his wishes. The clouds, indeed, seem sometimes to issue from the feet, and sometimes from the bowels, of these mountains, in passing the streaming sides of which the traveller is on the brightest day involved in the thickest mist; while the summit of the mountain above, and the valley below, are gilded by the sunbeams, which the vapours have not sullied.

The wild aspect of the country gives fresh horror and majesty to the grand pass of Pont Aberglasslyn; but in the midst of this sterile scene the beautiful vale of Festiniog, suddenly bursting on the sight, discloses the strong contrast of its charms. Reach Tan-y-bwlch, and tracing the valley to the little village of Festiniog, proceed

Page 488.

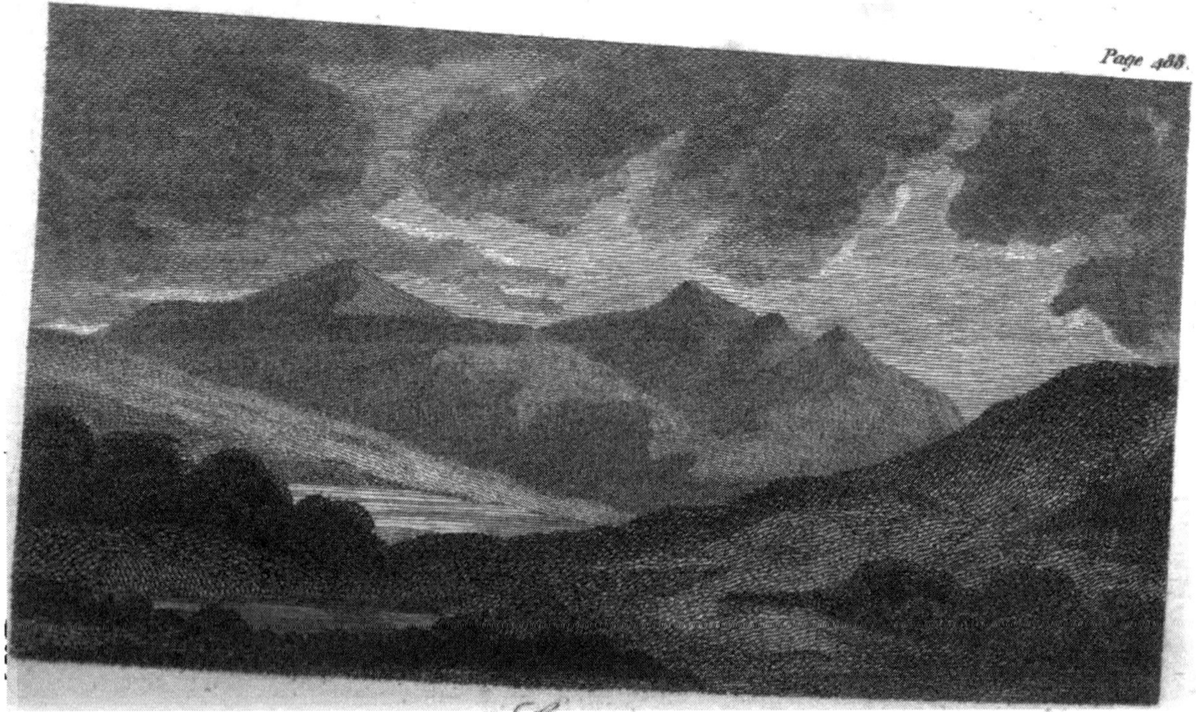

Snowdon.

to visit the Hall of Rhaidr-Du, lying in the recess of a narrow glen.

Harlech is the next object of attraction, to which the road lies over a chain of mountains. The castle is a noble edifice, and the most perfect of the fastnesses built by Edward I.

Pass the mean village of Trawsynnydo, and view the famous cascade of Dollymyllin.

Reach Dolgelly, the modern capital of Merioneth, a poor irregular place, standing under the northern base of Cader Idris, terminating in two peaks of unequal height.* This is one of the loftiest of the Welch mountains, the summit of which, like its famous rivals Snowden and Plinlimmon, is covered with entire snow, while numberless flocks of sheep, whose fleeces, bleached by the wind blowing fresh from the heavens, are scarcely less white than that snow, feed, frolick, and repose, on its ample sides. The eye aches to view the top of this mountain giant, and the brain turns dizzy as it surveys, by a sudden transition, the depth of the valley below.

Close to Dolgelly the Mawddach and Avon unite, and flow towards BARMOUTH, amidst the most picturesque scenery. This little sea-port consists of a single irregular street, only one side of which is built upon, and that on a solid rocky mountain, which is of so stupendous a height, that the first view of it, upon the traveller's entrance into the village, makes him not only tremble for himself, but for the aerial inhabitants! The houses are raised on terraces, above one another, in a very romantic style. Barmouth is much frequented, for the purpose of sea-bathing, and has several excellent machines.

Returning to Dolgelly, pursue the course of the Avon for some way; and, reaching the lake of Bala, or Pemble Meer, coast its north shore to the town of Bala, consisting principally of one handsome street. Here stands the elegant seat of Mr. Price.

Visit the pass of Glyndyffis, and soon reach Corwen on the Dee, the territory of Owen Glendower, the opponent of Henry IV.

* Cader Idris is 2850 feet above the level of Dolgelly Pier; and the great peak of Snowden is more than 3600 above the quay of Caernarvon.

Make a diversion to Llandisilio, the charming seat of Mr. Jones, and, in a narrow recess, come in sight of Valle Crucis Abbey, hemmed in on every side by chains of mountains, and fitted almost beyond every other place for monastic seclusion. Considerable fragments of it still remain.

Thence, tracing the banks of the Dee, advance to Llangollen, beautifully situate on the southern bank of that river, and almost surrounded by the Berwy mountains, the most extensive, though not the highest ridge in Wales. The vale of Llangollen is famous for its being the scene of the romantic friendship of two ladies of fashion. Their house and grounds are laid out with abundant taste, and have frequently been celebrated by the poet and tourist.

Cross the Berwyin to Llanrhaidr, and thence visit the grand cataract of Pishl-Rhaidr. Proceed to Llanvillyng, a small town of Montgomeryshire, and soon reach Welch-pool, one of the most flourishing towns in Wales. It stands in a fine vale, a little above the banks of the Severn, and close to the fine grounds of Powis Castle, a heavy but majestic pile.

Trace the valley, watered by the infant Severn, amidst populous towns and villages, to Newtown, and from thence proceed to Llanidloes, a town of some note, in the vicinity of which both the Severn and the Wye rise, at no great distance from each other, in the recesses of Plinlimmon, which towers in all its majesty.

Quitting the banks of the Severn, advance towards those of the Wye, and descend to that river, which is here uninteresting, at the melancholy village of Llangerig. The road is now carried over a narrow shelf of impending precipices, but soon descends to the banks of the Rhydol. Reach the village of Spwtty; and, passing beneath the woods of Hafod, descend to the banks of the Tivy, to visit the mouldering remains of Strata Florida Abbey.*

Pass Crosswood, the seat of lord Lisburne, to the ancient town of Llanbadern Vawr; and, taking Tallysont in the way, gain a view of the coast, and of the river and vale of Dovey, containing several populous villages and considerable iron works.

* See Aberystwith.

Cross the stream of Llysnant, which divides Montgomery from Cardigan, and soon reach the town of Machynthleth, a tolerably large place, situate on the Dovey. Proceed to the almost deserted town of Dinasmouthy, round which Nature assumes her rudest dress, and thence penetrate into the recesses of those heights in which the Dovey rises.

Re-enter Montgomeryshire at Malwydd, where is a remarkably large yew-tree; then, touching at the inn of Cann, reach the small town of Llainvair, agreeably situate in a deep hollow, surrounded by woody hills.

Pass Nantcribba, a pleasant seat of lord Hereford, and arrive at Montgomery, an indifferent town, but strikingly situated. The fragments of its castle exhibit a very picturesque appearance. At the distance of a few miles from this place re-enter England, and thus finish the Tour of North Wales, which every-where presents the most sublime and romantic scenery.

We deeply regret the circumscribed boundary we are constrained to observe, in our brief description of this lovely principality; the natural graces of which certainly claim pre-eminence on the score of romantic beauty, generally speaking, over any thing which the British empire has to offer. The most vivid descriptions of GILPIN, joined to those which have been given to the public by the sterling PENNANT, together with the fascinating sketches of PRATT, should only serve to excite curiosity to compare the original, to which no copy can do justice. To adopt the language of the latter writer, in a passage we borrow from his "Gleanings through Wales," and which shall close our account of the principality:—"The traveller who journeys into Wales should not be contented with any thing short of Nature's own volume, in every page of which she will present him with something to admire or imitate; something which, though admired and described before, will supply new description, new imitation; the beauties are often expanded from one shire to another, with succession both of the beautiful and sublime, and sometimes to the stretch of thirty or forty miles, in the progress of which, the fancy and the heart, the understanding, and all the higher emotions of the soul, are, by turns, regaled and delighted."

"In a word, whatever are the motives, habits, or character of a traveller, they would all be gratified in a tour through Wales, allowing time to do justice to nature and themselves; and, indeed, none but the most worthless or dissipated of human kind could observe, within the limits of a morning's ride or walk, such an assemblage of natural wonders, viewed at any period of the year, without tasting a pleasure of that moral kind, which, in looking above or below, must pronounce the objects of divine origin." "I have stood gazing (says Mr. Pratt) on some of these—Snowden and Plinlimmon, the vale of Cleyn, for instance, till they seemed of themselves to say, "Traveller! well mayest thou gaze; we merit your praises and admiration—we are of God!"

ITINERARY,

FROM

LONDON

TO THE

Mineral Water and Sea-Bathing Places,

DESCRIBED IN THIS GUIDE.

*** When the distances vary from those given in the body of the work, it must be presumed that a better or more frequented road has been adopted. The stages commence from the usual standards.

ROUTE I.

To ABERYSTWITH, through *Worcester.*

	M	M
Uxbridge - -		15
Beaconsfield -	8	23
High Wycombe	6	29
Tetsworth - -	13	42
OXFORD - - -	12	54
Woodstock - -	8	62
Enstone - - -	7	69
Chipping Norton	5	74
Moreton in Marsh	9	83
Broadway - -	8	91
Pershore - -	12	103
WORCESTER - -	9	112
Bromyard - -	14	126
Leominster - -	12	138
Presteigne - -	14	152
New Radnor -	7	159
Rhayader - -	18	177
Cwm-Ystwith -	14	191
Aberystwith -	16	207

To Aberystwith through Gloucester is somewhat more distant, and the roads are not so good.

ROUTE II.

To BATH and BRISTOL.

	M	M
Hounslow - -		10
Colnbrook - -	7	17
Slough - - -	3½	20½
Maidenhead -	5½	26
Reading - - -	13	39
Speenhamland - (Newbury)	16½	55½
Hungerford - -	8½	64
Marlborough -	10	74
Calne - - -	13	87
Chippenham -	6	93
BATH - - -	13	106
Keynsham - -	7½	113½
Brislington - -	3	116½
BRISTOL - - -	2½	119

Though this is the most frequented road, in point of distance it does not make above two or three miles difference, whether the traveller goes by Chippenham, or by

	M	M
Andover—by Devizes—by Sandy Lane—or by Windsor.		

ROUTE III.

To Blackpool.

	M	M
To Ashborn (see Buxton) Route VIII.		140
Leek - - - -	15	155
Macclesfield -	13	168
Stockport - -	11½	179½
Manchester - -	6½	186
West Houghton	13½	199½
Preston - - -	17½	217
Kirkham - -	9	226
Blackpool - -	8	234

ROUTE IV.

To Bognor.

	M	M
Kingston - -		12
Esher - - -	4	16
Ripley - - -	7½	23½
Guildford - -	6	30
Godalming - -	4	34
Haslemere - -	9	43
Midhurst - -	7½	50½
Chichester -	12½	62½
Bognor Hotel -	6½	69

ROUTE V.

To Bridlington Quay.

	M	M
Waltham Cross		11½
Ware - - -	9	20½
Buntingford -	10	30½
Royston -	7	37½
Arrington - -	6½	44
Huntingdon -	14½	58½
Stilton - - -	12½	71
Peterborough	6½	77½
Market-Deeping	9	86½
Bourn - -	7	93½
Folkingham -	9	102½
Sleaford - - -	9	111½
Lincoln - - -	17½	129
Spittal Inn - -	12	141
Brigg - - -	11	152
Barton - - -	11	163
Hull - - - -	7	170
Beverley - -	9	179
Great Driffield	13	192
Kilham - - -	5	197
Bridlington Quay	9	206

ROUTE VI.

To Brighton.

	M	M
Croydon - -		10
Godstone-Green	9½	19½
East Grinstead	9	28½
Uckfield - -	13	41½
Lewes - - -	8	49½
Brighton - -	8½	58

By Horsham and Steyning, the distance from London to Brighton is 61 miles. The following is the nearest route.

ROUTE VII.

To Brighton, by *Ryegate.*

	M	M
Sutton - - -		11
Ryegate - - -	9½	20½
Crawley - -	9½	30
Cuckfield - -	9½	39½
Brighton - -	14½	54

To Bristol. See Bath, Route II.

Broadstairs. See Margate.

ROUTE VIII.

To Buxton.

	M	M
Barnet - - -		11
St. Alban's - -	10	21
Dunstable - -	12½	33½
Newport Pagnel	18	51½
Northampton -	15	66½
Market Harbro'	17	83½
Leicester - -	14½	98
Loughborough	11½	109½
Derby - -	17	126½
Ashborn - - -	13½	140
Newhaven Inn	9	149
Hindlow House	4	153
Buxton - - -	6½	159½

The road to Buxton through Litchfield and Uttoxeter, is between 7 and 8 miles farther, nor does it, in general, pass through such an interesting country.

ROUTE IX.

To Cheltenham, by *Henley-on Thames.*

	M	M
Maidenhead. (See Route II) -		26
Henley-on-Thames	9	35
Benson - - -	11	46
Nuneham - -	6½	52
Oxford - - -	5½	58
Witney - - -	11	69
Burford - - -	7	76
Northleach - -	8	84
Frog-Mill - -	7	91
Cheltenham - -	6	97

The road to Cheltenham, through Woodstock and Chipping Norton, is only a very few miles round; and, as it gives the traveller an opportunity of seeing Blenheim, it is generally preferred.

To Cowes. (See Southampton.)

ROUTE X.

To Cromer.

	M	M
Epping - - -		16½
Harlowe . -	7	23½
Sawbridgeworth	2	25½
Bishops-Stortford	4½	30
Quendon	6	36
Great Chesterford	8½	44½
Newmarket -	16½	61
Thetford - -	19	80
Attleburgh - -	14	94
Hetherset - -	9½	103½
Norwich - -	5½	109
North Walsham	15	124
Cromer - - -	9	133

Taking the road by Bury, or by Ipswich, to Norwich, the distance to Cromer will be a few miles greater, and by proceeding thro' East Dereham instead of North Walsham, it will be reduced about three miles.

ROUTE XI.

To Dover.

	M	M
Dartford - -		15

	M	M
Northfleet - -	5½	20½
Rochester - -	9	29½
Sittingbourn -	11	40½
Ospringe - -	6	46½
Canterbury - -	9	55½
Half-way House	7½	63
Dover	8	71

To Dawlish. (See Teignmouth.)

ROUTE XII.

To East-Bourne.

Bromley - -		10
Seven Oaks - -	13½	23½
Tunbridge - -	6½	30
Tunbridge Wells	6	36
Cross-in-Hand -	12	48
East-Bourne	14½	62½

There is another road to East Bourne, through Uckfield, by which upwards of two miles are saved.

ROUTE XIII.

To Exmouth.

To Charmouth (see Route XXII.)		141
Colyford - -	9	150
Sidmouth - -	9	159
Otterton - -	3	162½
Exmouth - -	6	168½

ROUTE XIV.

To Folkestone.

To Canterbury (see Route XI.) -		55½
Bridge - - -	3	58½
Folkestone . -	15½	74

ROUTE XV.

To Fowey.

	M	M
To Charmouth (see Route XXII.)		141
Axminster - -	5½	146½
Honiton - -	9½	156
Exeter - - -	16½	172½
Chudleigh - -	9½	182
Ashburton - -	9½	191½
Ivy Bridge - -	13	204½
Plymouth Dock	13	217½
Cross the Tamer to Crofthole - -	6	223½
East Looe - -	7½	231
Fowey - - -	8	239

ROUTE XVI.

To Harrowgate.

Loughborough (Route VIII.)		109½
Nottingham	15½	125
Mansfield - -	14	139
Chesterfield -	12½	151½
Sheffield - - -	12½	164
Barnsley - -	13½	177½
Wakefield - -	10	187½
Leeds - - -	9	196½
Harewood - -	8	204½
Harrowgate -	7	211½

Travellers, who wish to visit Oxford, may proceed by Birmingham, through Ashby-de-la-Zouch, to Nottingham, and then fall into the preceding road.

ROUTE XVII.

To Harwich.

Romford - -		12

	M	M
Brentwood - -	6	18
Chelmsford - -	11	29
Kelvedon - -	12	41
Colchester - -	10	51
Bradfield - -	12	63
Harwich - -	8½	71½

ROUTE XVIII.

To HASTINGS.

	M	M
Tunbridge Wells (Route XII.)		36
Hurst Green -	13½	49½
Hastings - -	16	65½

ROUTE XIX.

To ILFRACOMBE.

	M	M
Brentford - -		7
Staines - - -	9	16
Bagshot - - -	10	26
Blackwater -	4	30
Basingstoke -	15	45
Whitchurch -	11½	56½
Andover - -	7	63½
Amesbury - -	14	77½
Deptford Inn -	9½	87
Mere - - - - -	14	101
Wincanton - -	7	108
Somerton - -	17½	125½
Taunton - - -	19	144½
Wellington - -	7	151½
Tiverton - - -	14	165½
South Molton -	18½	184
Barnstaple - -	11½	195½
Ilfracombe - -	10	205½

To LYMINGTON. (See Route XXVIII. to SOUTHAMPTON.)

ROUTE XX.

To LEMINGTON PRIORS.

	M	M
Barnet - - -		11
St. Albans - -	10	21
Dunstable - -	12½	33½
Stony Stratford	19½	53
Towcester - -	7½	60½
Daventry - -	12	72½
Southam - - -	10½	83
Lemington Priors	7	90

ROUTE XXI.

To LITTLE HAMPTON.

	M	M
Epsom - - -		14
Dorking - - -	9	23
Kingfold - -	9	32
Slinfold - - -	6	38
Pulborough - -	10	48
Arundel - - -	9	57
Little Hampton	4	61

ROUTE XXII.

To LYME-REGIS and CHARMOUTH.

	M	M
Andover. (See Route XV.) -		63
SALISBURY - -	17½	80½
Woodyates Inn	10½	91
Blandford - -	12	103
Dorchester - -	16	119
Bridport - -	15½	134
Charmouth - -	7	141
Lyme-Regis -	2½	143½

ROUTE XXIII.

To MALVERN.

	M	M
Worcester. (See Route I.) -		112
Malvern - - -	8	119

ROUTE XXIV.

To MARGATE.

	M	M
Dartford - -		15
Rochester - -	14	29
Sittingbourne -	11	40
CANTERBURY -	15½	55½
Upseet - -	6	61½
Monkton - -	5	66½
Margate - -	5½	72

Three miles south-east of Margate, and two north from Ramsgate, stands the fashionable village of Broadstairs.

ROUTE XXV.

To MATLOCK.

	M	M
Derby (Route VIII.) - -		126
Sandyford - -	10	136
Matlock - - -	7½	143½

There is another road to Matlock, through Wirksworth, which increases the distance about a mile.

ROUTE XXVI.

To RAMSGATE.

	M	M
CANTERBURY (Route XI.)		55
Monkton - -	11½	66½
Ramsgate - -	7	73½

ROUTE XXVII.

To SCARBOROUGH.

	M	M
To Great Driffield (See Route V.)		192
Scarborough -	22	214

To SIDMOUTH. (See Route XIII. to Exmouth.)

ROUTE XXVIII.

To SOUTHAMPTON.

	M	M
Bagshot (See Route XIX.)		26
Farnham - -	12	38
Alton - - -	9	47
Alresford - -	10	57
WINCHESTER -	8	65
Southampton -	12	77

Eighteen miles from Southampton, thro' Lyndhurst, which is half way, stands Lymington.

Between Southampton and Cowes, in the Isle of Wight, by the packet, is 16 miles. (See the Tour of the Isle of Wight.)

ROUTE XXIX.

To SOUTHEND.

	M	M
Brentwood (Route XVII.) - -		18
Billericay - -	5	23
Raleigh - - -	10½	33½
Southend - -	9	42½

ROUTE XXX.

To SWANSEA.

	M	M
BRISTOL. (See Route II.) -		119
New Passage -	10½	129½
Caerwent - -	6½	136

	M	M
Newport - -	11	147
Cardiff - - -	12½	159½
Cowbridge - -	12½	172
Pyle - - - -	13	185
Neath - - -	12	197
Swansea - -	9	206

From hence, by Carmarthen and St. Clare, is a road to Tenby, as much frequented as Route XXXII.

ROUTE XXXI.

To TEIGNMOUTH and SHALDON.

Charmouth (Route XXII.) - - -		141
Axminster - -	6	147
Honiton - - -	9½	156½
EXETER - - -	16½	173
Alphington - -	1½	174½
Haldon - - -	4	178½
Teignmouth - -	8½	187

Dawlish lies about the same distance from London as Teignmouth; from the latter, it is only three miles.

A ferry across the Teign connects Shaldon and Teignmouth.

ROUTE XXXII.

To TENBY.

Oxford, by Wycombe (Route I.)		54
Witney - - -	11	65
Burford - - -	8	73
Northleach - -	9	82
Cheltenham - -	12½	94½
GLOUCESTER -	9½	104
Ross - - - -	16½	120½
Monmouth - -	10½	131
Abergavenny -	17	148
Crickhowel - -	6	154
Brecon - - -	14	168
Llandovery - -	20	188
Llandilo-Vawr -	14½	202½
Caermarthen -	15½	218
Tavernspite - -	16½	234½
Tenby - - - -	9½	244

For another road to Tenby, see XXX.

ROUTE XXXIII.

To TUNBRIDGE-WELLS.

(See Route XII.)

There are several roads to Tunbridge-Wells. That through Penshurst makes the distance from London thirty-seven miles.

ROUTE XXXIV.

To WEYMOUTH.

Dorchester (Route XXII.) - -		120
Broadway - -	5	125
Weymouth - -	3	128

ROUTE XXXV.

To WORTHING.

Dorking (See Route XXI.) - - -		23
Horsham - - -	13	36
Ashington - -	10	46
Worthing - -	8	54

The old road by Steyning is longer by two miles, and incommodious on account of the hills.

ROUTE XXXVI.

To YARMOUTH.

	M.	M.
Colchester (Route XVII.) -		51
Ipswich - - - -	18	69
Woodbridge - -	8	77
Saxmundham -	12½	89½
Wrangford - -	12½	102
Lowestoff - -	11½	113½
Yarmouth - -	10	123½

Correct Itinerary of a Tour round the South Coast of ENGLAND, from *Margate* to *Teignmouth*, including a distance of Two Hundred and Forty Miles, and many of the principal Sea-Bathing Places.

	M.
Kingsgate - - -	2¾
North Foreland Light-House - - - -	3½
BROADSTAIRS - -	4¾
RAMSGATE - - -	6¾
St. Lawrence - -	7½
SANDWICH - - -	12¼
DEAL - - - - - -	17¼
Walmer Castle - -	18¾
South Foreland to the left.	
Westley - - - -	22¾
DOVER - - - -	26¼
The French coast visible from the heights. A fine view before the descent to Folkestone.	
FOLKESTONE - - -	33¼
SANDGATE - - -	35¼
HYTHE - - - -	37¼
Dimchurch - - -	43
NEW ROMNEY - -	47
Dungeness, to the South; Boulogne exactly opposite, on the French Coast.	
Old Romney - -	49
Cross the Marshes -	
RYE - - - - - -	58
WINCHELSEA - - -	61
HASTINGS (only one Inn) - - - -	63
Beachy head now becomes a grand prominence to the South-West.	
Bexhill - - - -	75
Pevensey Bay - -	83
Here William the Conqueror landed.	
EAST BOURNE - -	88½
SEAFORD - - - -	96½
Newhaven - - -	100
Rottingdean - - -	105
BRIGHTON - - -	[illegible]
Shoreham - - -	116
Leave Worthing to the left.	
ARUNDEL - - - -	[illegible]
The Castle is worth seeing.	
Crocker Hill - -	[illegible]
Leave Bognor and Selsey Bill on the left.	
[illegible]	[illegible]
CHICHESTER - - -	[illegible]

	M.
Nutbourn - - -	143½
Havant - - - -	147½
Cosham - - - -	151¾
Hilsea - - - -	153
PORTSMOUTH - -	156½

The dock-yards and harbour deserve notice. The best inns are the Crown, George, Fountain, and Navy Tavern.

	M.
GOSPORT - - - -	157
FAREHAM - - -	162
Wickham - - -	165¼
Bottley - - - -	170
Swathling - - -	175½
SOUTHAMPTON - -	179
Redbridge - - -	182½
LYNDHURST - - -	188½
LYMINGTON - - -	196¼
Milton Green - -	203
CHRIST CHURCH - -	208
Kingston - - - -	215¾
POOLE - - - - -	221¾
Ditchett - - - -	228

	M.
WAREHAM - - -	234
Wemrith - - - -	243
Warmwell - - -	248

Portland Island to the left, stretches nearly 10 miles into the sea.

	M.
Preston - - - -	253
Melcombe Regis -	255
WEYMOUTH - - -	256
Brodeway - - -	261
Winterborne St. Martins - - - - -	267
BRIDPORT - - -	279
Charmouth - - -	286
LYME REGIS - - -	288
Colyford - - - -	294½
SIDMOUTH - - -	304½
Otterton - - - -	308
EXMOUTH - - -	314
TOPSHAM - - - -	321
EXETER - - - -	326
Kenford - - - -	330
Haldon - - - -	332
Teignmouth - - -	341

A Tour round the Welch Coast from Gloucester, by Milford Haven and Aberystwith, to Chester.

	M.
To Tenby (See Route XXXII.) *from Gloucester* - - - -	140
Pembroke - - - -	150
The Ferry - - -	152
Haverford West -	159
Ryston Mountain -	162
Cornellach - - -	168
New Inn - - - -	171
Poutbrynbarden -	175
Eglwysorw - - -	179
Cardigan - - - -	185
Blaneport - - -	191

	M.
New Inn - - - -	196
Llanarth - - - -	203
Morva - - - -	215
Llanrhysted - - -	219
Ridalvin - - - -	226
Aberystwith - - -	228
Tal-y-bont - - -	235
Garreg - - - -	241
Machynleth - - -	246

Plynlimmon to the right. and Cader Idris to the left

	M.
Cemmes - - - -	248

	M.		M.
Dinas-mouthy - -	258	*Bangor* - - - - -	314
Dolgelly - - - -	267	Aber - - - - - -	320
Trawsvynid - - -	278	Penmanmawr - -	323
Tan-y-bwlch - -	284	Aberconway - -	329
		Abergeley - - -	341
Snowden to the right.		St. Asaph - - - - -	348
Aberglaslyn Bridge	291	*Holywell* - - - -	358
Bettws - - - -	299	Northop - - - - -	364
Caernarvon - - -	305	Hawarden - - -	369
Llanfairscar - - -	308	*Chester* - - - - -	375

OBSERVATIONS

ON

Mineral Waters, and on Sea-Bathing,

WITH

CAUTIONS AND ADMONITIONS

ON THEIR

USE AND APPLICATION.

IN the course of the foregoing work will be found an analysis of the different mineral waters, visited, with an enumeration of their qualities and effects; but as it may be satisfactory to know the principal component parts and classification of those salutary springs in general, we borrow the arrangement and remarks of the learned and ingenious Dr. THOMSON, in his late excellent work, "*The Family Physician,*" on this subject; premising, that some medical person on the spot should always be consulted, in regard to the use and application of every kind of mineral water.

"The various substances," says this able writer, "occasionally found united with water, may be comprised chiefly under four classes; aerial, saline, metal' c, and earthy.

"The first of these classes contains atmospheric, vital, fixed, inflammable, hepatic, and phlogisticated airs.

"The second contains vitriolic, nitrous, and marine acids; natron, kali, ammonia, and sulphurated kali.

"The third contains iron, copper, zinc, manganese, and arsenic.

"The fourth contains magnesia, lime, clay, barytes, and siliceous earth.

"Of neutral salts, the vitriolic acid is found united with natron, kali, lime, magnesia, clay, iron, copper, and zinc.

"The nitrous acid, with the four former of these. The marine acid with the same, and sometimes with barytes, manganese, and clay. And the aerial acid with these, and also with iron, zinc, and manganese.

"Sulphur, fossile oil, and extracts from vegetable and animal substances, are also found sometimes in mineral waters.

"From the various substances above-mentioned, and their different combinations, are derived all the virtues of mineral waters, except such as they obtain from their temperature.

CLASSIFICATION OF MINERAL WATERS.

CHALYBEATE WATERS.

Of all the mineral waters, the chalybeate are the class most useful and beneficial to health; and are very plentiful in this island.

Waters are known to be chalybeate by their striking a reddish purple, or black colour, with an infusion of galls; and according to the height of the colour, provided the strength of the infusion be the same, we invariably judge of the strength of the water as a chalybeate.

The iron in these waters is held in solution by means of fixed air; and as this flies off on exposing the water, the iron falls to the bottom, in form of a brownish yellow powder. Hence these waters strike the deepest black with galls, at the spring head; and in time they wholly lose that property. They have a brisk, acidulous, or vinous taste, when fresh, and tinge the stools black.

Chalybeate waters, taken inwardly, strengthen the constitution in general, increase the tone of the fibres, quicken the circulation, and restore a proper consistence to the blood when in a too thin and watery state. Hence they are good in diseases arising from weakness; in spasmodic disorders, arising from too great irritability and relaxation of the nervous system; in fluor albus, and gleets; in female obstructions; in hysteric and hypochondriacal disorders; in loss of appetite and indigestion; and in a variety of other complaints, dependent on a weak state of body.

Though mineral waters, in general, should never be resorted to without medical advice, it may be here proper to observe, that previous to a course of chalybeate waters, bleeding, and a cooling purge, may be necessary, in case of heat, and any disposition to fever. Indeed, where there is much fever, and also in ulcers of the lungs, and in confirmed obstructions attended with fever, the use of these waters is improper. It is also a necessary caution, that costiveness should be avoided while drinking them.

Patients ought to begin by drinking a small quantity of these waters every morning, and gradually increase the dose. A temperate diet, and gentle exercise, should always be observed while taking them.

If the water should prove too cold, a bottle containing some of it may be placed in warm water just before drinking.

Acids, tea, and other things which decompose those waters, should not be taken for some time before or after drinking them.

Besides iron, these waters usually contain sea-salt, natron, a purging salt, and other substances.

CHALYBEATE PURGING WATERS.

Chalybeate Purging Waters contain a greater proportion of purging-salt than of any other solid matter, and therefore when taken in sufficient quantity, or that of several pints, they operate by stool. They have this advantage over other purges, that they do not exhaust the strength.

If taken in less quantity, as alteratives, they operate chiefly by urine. The principal of this class are

SULPHUREOUS WATERS.

Sulphureous Waters, though so named, do not contain an actual sulphur, but are impregnated with a gas, or subtle spirit, which gives them their sulphureous smell. Besides this, they usually contain either natron, sea-salt, a purging salt, iron, earth, or other matter, and commonly several of these in different proportions.

Waters of this sort are diuretic, and strongly diaphoretic, and are therefore good in cutaneous diseases, used both internally and externally. They are also good in chronic obstructions, and in disorders proceeding from acidity, worms, &c. They usually make silver appear of a copper colour.

SULPHUREOUS PURGING WATERS.

Sulphureous purging Waters differ from the preceding in containing a purging salt as the principal solid ingredient, and therefore operating by stool. They are good in the same disorders as the alterative sulphureous waters, as also for foulness of the bowels, &c.

SALINE WATERS.

Acidulous, or *saline waters*, contain natron. This salt, as the waters are taken up from the fountain, is saturate, or rather supersaturate, with fixed air; hence the waters do not then manifest any alkaline quality; on the contrary, they curdle with soap, and are termed *acidulæ*. This fixed air, or aeriel acid, however, being very volatile, soon exhales when the water is heated, or stands a while exposed, and then the alkali manifests itself.

The operation of these waters is chiefly by urine, for they have little or no purgative virtue. They serve to correct acidities, render the blood and juices more fluid, and promotes a brisk and free circulation. Hence they are good in obstructions of the glands, and against gross and viscid humours. They are useful in the gravel and stone, and in other disorders of the kidneys and bladder, as well as in gouty and rheumatic complaints, cutaneous disorders, and likewise those of the nervous kind.

VITRIOLIC WATERS.

Vitriolic Waters are those which are impregnated with green vitriol or copperas, and strike a black colour with galls. They are chiefly used externally for washing old sores and the like, and frequently with good effect. In some cases, however, they are taken inwardly in small doses, and then they prove emetic and purgative.

HOT MINERAL WATERS.

There are in England a great number of *cold* mineral waters; but of the *hot* very few.

The *warm* waters possess many of the virtues and properties of *cold* waters of the same class, and which are impregnated in the same manner; but they are preferable in many cases, as from their warmth they are more kindly and agreeable to the stomachs of weak people, and promote perspiration.

The warm waters are also used as warm baths, and may in general be considered as warm medicated baths. By relaxing the fibres, they are useful in a variety of disorders which arise from rigidity, and spasm, and also from other causes. Hence they are of great use in rheumatisms, inflammations, costiveness, &c. in which the cure is commonly assisted by the internal use of those waters.

SEA-BATHING.

On the subject of bathing, particularly in salt water, much has been written by medical men; but as no general rules can apply to individual cases, what has been said in regard to drinking mineral waters equally applies here too, that the advice of a physician should always be taken before a valetudinarian commences a course of bathing, either in fresh or salt, hot or cold water.

The general and indiscriminate use of bathing is allowed on all hands, frequently to lay the foundation of a train of maladies, and instead of being a harmless or salutary amusement, is often destructive to health and enjoyment.

In order to secure the good effects of cold bathing, a previous immersion or two in a tepid bath, of about eighty-four, will be highly conducive. The body will thus be purified, and the absorbent vessels will have an opportunity of acting with more freedom and force.

Bathing early in the morning, is, in many respects, preferable to a late hour, when the constitution is able to bear it. It induces a habit of early rising, and the water at that period of the day, being most cool, of consequence has a more tonic effect.

They who bathe every morning, instead of strengthening the habit, take the surest way to weaken it. Twice or thrice in a week is amply sufficient; and instead of continuing long in the water, or taking repeated dips, the first plunge is the only one that can be attended with any utility.

At the commencement of a course of bathing, twice a week is enough; and thrice in the middle. Before its close, the bather should again confine himself to an immersion every three days, or even at a longer interval.

Salt water, even if not thoroughly wiped from the body, is not apt to give cold, and therefore the bather, after an immersion, need not be anxious on this account; but proceed to take such exercise as may keep up moderately, or promote the salutary glow, which is the test of the bath agreeing with the constitution. Fatigue should be avoided by those who have recourse to the cold water for debility; their own feelings will be the best direction.

N.B. The Communication of Corrections and necessary Additions, and the Loan of correct Drawings, will be thankfully acknowledged.

A TABLE of the relative Distances, by

N. B. *To find the Distance from any one Place to another last in Alphabetical Order look down the Side. Whe look along the Top for Brighton,*

	LONDON	Aberystwith	Bath	Bognor	Brighton	Bristol	Broadstairs
Aberystwith	210						
Bath	106	135					
Bognor	69	230	98				
Brighton	54	185	117	25			
Bristol	118	122	12	110	138		
Broadstairs	76	272	180	135	89	186	
Buxton	160	140	150	210	222	159	218
Cheltenham	95	110	47	118	140	43	167
Cromer	130	280	220	190	186	225	203
East Bourne	63	250	132	42	22	156	84
Harrowgate	212	203	223	254	256	217	269
Hastings	64	254	177	70	39	180	56
Lakes (Kendal)	262	202	248	305	317	240	333
Lyme Regis	143	175	69	108	137	68	217
Lymington	95	194	81	38	60	99	161
Malvern	120	96	58	134	166	54	180
Margate	73	271	180	132	90	187	3
Matlock	143	150	140	180	196	142	216
Ramsgate	74	270	177	129	86	184	2
Scarborough	214	258	274	281	276	276	287
Southend	44	260	152	110	102	161	117
Southampton	77	193	63	31	74	79	154
Swansea	206	64	69	190	218	79	275
Teignmouth	187	200	90	160	192	86	255
Tenby	244	80	142	235	266	130	313
Tunbridge Wells	37	250	143	54	30	150	65
Weymouth	128	187	67	95	122	65	205
Worthing	59	180	112	15	[illegible]	[illegible]	[illegible]

INDEX.

Directions for placing the Plates and Maps.

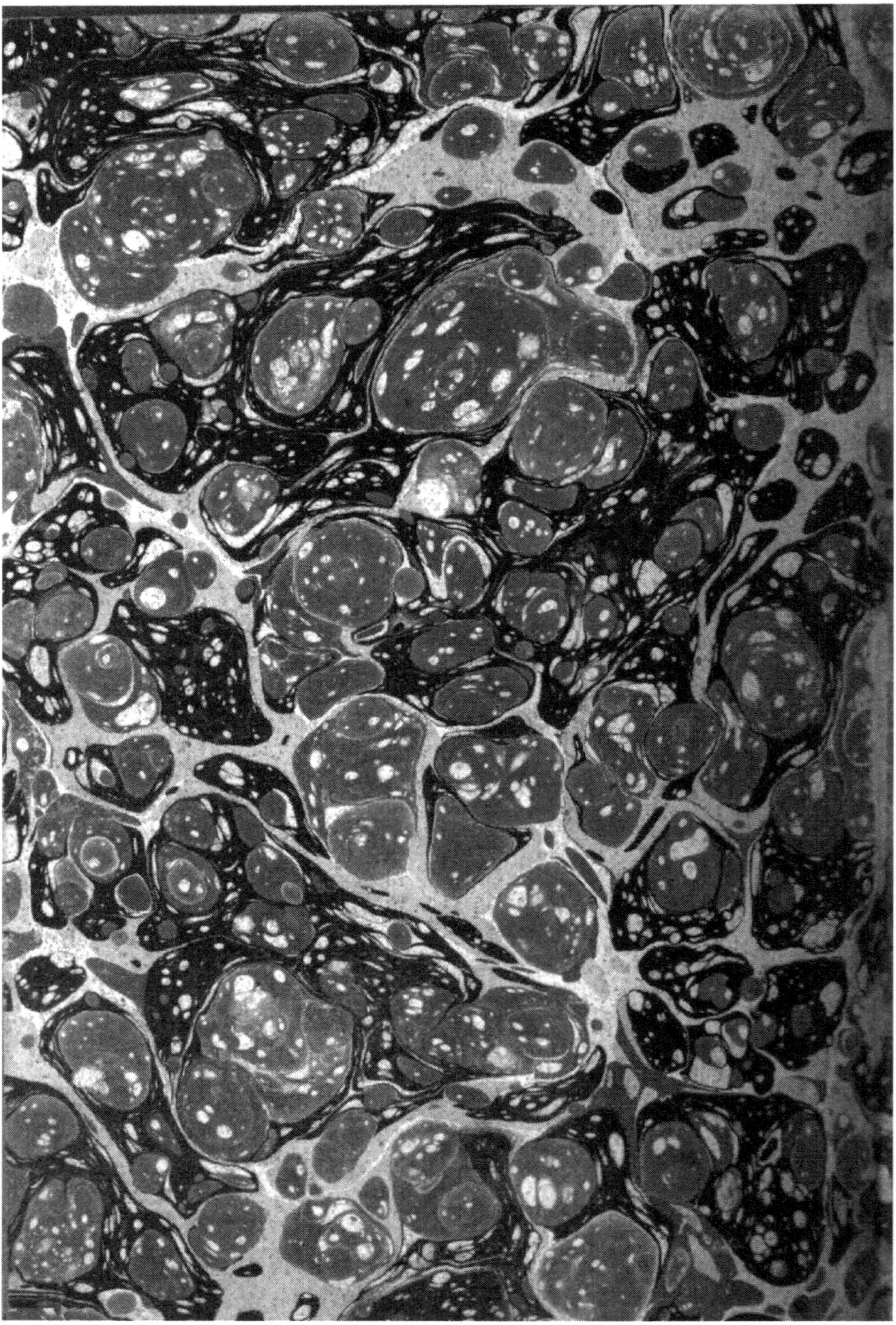

Milton Keynes UK
Ingram Content Group UK Ltd.
UKHW010832010224
437095UK00005B/259

9 781015 925649